KU-222-878

369 0294262

The Modernization of the Nursing Workforce

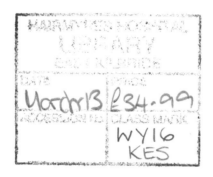

NORWICH HOSPITAL
LIBRARY
GREAT OLDEN

DATE	PRICE
March 13	£34.99
ACCESSION No.	CLASS MARK
	WY16 KES

The Modernization of the Nursing Workforce
Valuing the healthcare assistant

Ian Kessler
Reader in Employment Relations, Said Business School,
University of Oxford, Oxford, UK

Paul Heron
Senior Research Associate, Said Business School,
University of Oxford, Oxford, UK

Sue Dopson
Said Business School and Fellow of Green Templeton,
University of Oxford, Oxford, UK

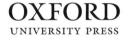

OXFORD
UNIVERSITY PRESS

OXFORD
UNIVERSITY PRESS

Great Clarendon Street, Oxford, OX2 6DP,
United Kingdom

Oxford University Press is a department of the University of Oxford.
It furthers the University's objective of excellence in research, scholarship,
and education by publishing worldwide. Oxford is a registered trade mark of
Oxford University Press in the UK and in certain other countries

© Oxford University Press 2012

Materials in chapters 1–10 reproduced with permission of the NIHR Service Delivery
Organisation programme Project ref: 08/1619/155. © Queen's Printer and Controller of
HMSO 2010. This work was produced by Kessler et al. under the terms of a
commissioning contract issued by the Secretary of State for Health.

The moral rights of the authors have been asserted

First Edition published in 2012

Impression: 1

All rights reserved. No part of this publication may be reproduced, stored in
a retrieval system, or transmitted, in any form or by any means, without the
prior permission in writing of Oxford University Press, or as expressly permitted
by law, by licence or under terms agreed with the appropriate reprographics
rights organization. Enquiries concerning reproduction outside the scope of the
above should be sent to the Rights Department, Oxford University Press, at the
address above

You must not circulate this work in any other form
and you must impose this same condition on any acquirer

British Library Cataloguing in Publication Data
Data available

Library of Congress Cataloging in Publication Data
Data available

ISBN 978–0–19–969413–6

Printed and bound by
CPI Group (UK) Ltd, Croydon, CR0 4YY

Oxford University Press makes no representation, express or implied, that the
drug dosages in this book are correct. Readers must therefore always check
the product information and clinical procedures with the most up-to-date
published product information and data sheets provided by the manufacturers
and the most recent codes of conduct and safety regulations. The authors and
the publishers do not accept responsibility or legal liability for any errors in the
text or for the misuse or misapplication of material in this work. Except where
otherwise stated, drug dosages and recommendations are for the non-pregnant
adult who is not breast-feeding

Links to third party websites are provided by Oxford in good faith and
for information only. Oxford disclaims any responsibility for the materials
contained in any third party website referenced in this work.

Preface

This book on nurse support workers in secondary healthcare reflects the authors' research interests developed over a considerable period of time. We have spent many years researching work and employment in publicly owned and run services: in social care, in education, in central government, and especially in the British National Health Service. We have also established a research engagement with public service workers in the lower reaches of the organizational hierarchy. These are workers often found on the less secure margins of the labour market, with a paucity of formal qualifications, sometimes from ethnic minority backgrounds, often presented with few social and economic opportunities during their working and personal lives.

More specifically, we have been attracted to the study of support workers in the public services, those working alongside, often assisting the professional. The rationale for this attraction is threefold. First there has, over recent years and particularly in the context of public service reform, been a proliferation of such support workers. Second, assistants are a group of workers who 'plough their trade' often unseen or overlooked by senior management and service users, despite being crucial to the functioning and well-being of the organization and its clients. Third, this is a group which generates a range of intriguing research questions. Drawn from the margins of the labour market, assistants are unregulated workers, usually working alongside the most skilled of work groups, the professional—the teacher, nurse and doctor, and the social worker—and directly dealing with the most vulnerable members of the community—the very young, the old, sick, and the excluded. What does the assistant bring to these situations? What are the costs and benefits derived from this unlikely workplace juxtaposition of the 'less skilled', the 'most capable', and the highly vulnerable?

Between 2003–2005 two of the authors, Ian Kessler and Paul Heron, embarked with Stephen Bach (King's College, University of London) on a two-year Economic and Social Research Council funded project looking at assistants in health, education, and social care. The research reported in this book developed from this earlier work, the National Institute for Health Research Service Delivery and Organisation (NIHR) supporting a more focused three-year study of healthcare assistants (HCAs) between 2007–2010. It is work which the NIHR has continued to fund in a follow-up project on HCAs running from 2011–2013.

Our work on assistants in the public services, and especially in the health service, has been characterized by a number of features. First, it has been policy driven: HCAs have been crucial to workforce developments in healthcare, and our research has sought to interrogate the assumptions upon which this policy has been based and provide a firmer foundation for future policy deliberations. Second, our research is unashamedly empiricist. Certainly, we have been keen to connect to analytical and theoretical debates, but our primary interest has been in generating rich empirical data to inform these debates. Third, our research has sought to engage: more specifically we have throughout been concerned to involve healthcare organizations and relevant actors at national, regional, and Trust levels, and feed back our findings in ways which they might find worthwhile and useful.

Given the nature of the study, our engagement with HCAs has been particularly close: we have spoken to hundreds of HCAs and spent many hours observing them at work. It is difficult not to be immensely impressed by the dedication and hard work of HCAs, responsible for the care of the most acutely sick in our society. One of the book's key aims is to connect the reader to the working lives of HCAs, and as a means of doing so considerable space has been devoted in this book to the unmediated voice of the HCA.

Of course, there is always the danger of case study researchers 'going native', but being deeply engaged with your research subject does not necessarily mean compromising scholarly and research standards. Indeed, the final characteristic of our work has been a commitment to a robust research approach: the case studies presented in this book have been based on a variety of research methods designed to generate a wealth of qualitative and quantitative data. This has enabled us to capture the perspective not only of HCAs, but also of the nurses they work with and the patients they care for.

We would not have been able to conduct research on this scale without the support of many individuals and groups. We would like to thank the many HCAs, nurses, patients, and hospital managers who gave their time and help to us, as research subjects and as organizers. We would like to give special thanks to Gail Adams from UNISON and Tanis Hand from the Royal College of Nursing (RCN): they remained interested in and supportive of our work. Special thanks are also due to Kerstin Helminger, who undertook some important additional, background research work for this book. We would also like to thank the members of our advisory group who provided invaluable advice as the project progressed (institutions are those which members represented during their time on the advisory group):

- Stephen Bach, King's College London;
- Roswyn Hakesley-Brown, Patients Association;

- Tony Halton, Department of Health;
- Ros Moore, Department of Health;
- Jane Naish, RCN;
- Jim O'Connell, NHS South Central;
- Deborah O'Dea, Healthcare People Management Association;
- Chris Pearson, Skills for Health;
- Jo Rycroft-Malone, RCN Institute;
- Lynda Scott, NHS Employers;
- Karen Spilsbury, University of York.

Thanks to the NIHR for funding this project and our follow-up work.

Research instruments used in this study—topic guides, interview schedules and questionnaires—are available on request.

Contents

Glossary of terms and abbreviations

Abbreviation	Term in full	Explanation of term
Trust	Acute Trust	Also known as an NHS hospital Trust, provides secondary health services within the NHS and is commissioned to provide these services by NHS primary care trusts
AfC	Agenda for Change	The 2004 collective agreement which established the current NHS grading and pay system for NHS staff. It harmonizes their pay scales and career progression arrangements across traditionally separate pay groups. There are nine new numbered pay bands subdivided into points, similar to the old alphabetic Whitley Council 'grades' pay scales
AP	Assistant Practitioner	A higher-level support worker at Agenda for Change pay band 4
BM	Blood monitoring	A routine and regular test to measure sugar levels within the blood
CQC	Care Quality Commission	Formerly the Healthcare Commission, it is a non-departmental public body established in 2009 to regulate and inspect health and social care services in England
DH	Department of Health	The department of the United Kingdom government with responsibility for government policy for England on health, social care and the National Health Service
FT	Foundation Trust	An NHS Trust that is part of the National Health Service in England and has gained a degree of independence from the Department of Health and local NHS strategic health authority
HCA	Healthcare Assistant	Nursing support role
HSW	Healthcare Support Worker	The more common job title for a nursing support role in Scotland
KSF	Knowledge and Skills Framework	A competence framework to support personal development and career progression within the NHS, introduced as part of Agenda for Change

Abbreviation	Term in full	Explanation of term
	Last Offices	The cleaning of the body and the laying out of the deceased for potential view by friends and relatives
MNC	Modernising Nursing Careers	Public Policy attempt to reorder and restructure nursing careers
NMC	Nursing and Midwifery Council	The body set up by Parliament to regulate the nurse and midwifery professions
NHS	National Health Service	The publicly-funded healthcare system in England
NVQ	National Vocation Qualification	Work based awards in England, Wales and Northern Ireland that are achieved through assessment and training
PDR	Performance Development Review	Integral to KSF, the approach for assessing individual performance.
	Project 2000	A scheme, introduced in 1989, that formed the basis for the academic education of all nurses and midwives.
QCF	Qualification and Credit Framework	New accreditation system for vocational qualifications
RCN	Royal College of Nursing	A membership organization representing nurses and nursing
	Secondary Healthcare	The service provided by medical specialists who generally do not have first contact with patients. The term is usually synonymous with 'hospital care'
SEN	State Enrolled Nurse	Prior to the implementation of Project 2000, SEN students used to follow the first 12 months training of the state registered nurses (SRNs, now known as level one nurses), and then had another 12 months of training before sitting SEN exams and becoming registered nurses
SHA	Strategic Health Authority	There are ten SHAs which form part of the structure of the National Health Service in England. Each SHA is responsible for enacting the directives and implementing fiscal policy as dictated by the Department of Health at a regional level
UNISON	UNISON	The main union representing support workers in healthcare

Introduction

Over recent years, the provision of healthcare in developed and less developed nations has faced a range of pressures as it seeks to address new demands and expectations, often in the context of a constrained or shrinking resource base. These pressures have inevitably focused attention on the structure and nature of the nursing workforce: how might this workforce be efficiently and effectively organized, developed, and managed to meet these upcoming challenges? It is a question which, in turn, has heightened interest in the nurse support role. In many countries this role has been a long-standing and an integral part of the nursing workforce. However, policymakers and practitioners have increasingly come to view the nurse support role as central to the pursuit of a variety of service and other organizational objectives. This heightened attention has placed the role under intense critical scrutiny, apparent in public policy debates on its implications for patient care and, more specifically, on whether and how it might be regulated (Department of Health, 2004). In short, despite, or more plausibly because of, its increasing importance to nursing and healthcare provision, the support role has been subject to increasing challenge and concern within the public domain.

These debates have been conducted on a remarkably weak evidence base on the nature and consequences of the nurse support role. For example, public policymaker and practitioner aspirations have often been founded on heroic, largely untested, assumptions about the capacity of the role and those who perform it to contribute through 'new' and 'better' ways of working. Indeed, despite increased general interest in the role, knowledge about its character and impact remains fragmented and patchy. This knowledge gap has been long-standing, memorably encapsulated almost fifteen years ago when Carole Thornley referred to healthcare assistants (HCAs) as 'invisible workers'.

This book aims to deepen our understanding of the nurse support role in an acute healthcare setting, with a view to establishing a firmer foundation for policymakers and practitioners to develop and manage it.

As implied, the focus of this book is a role which works alongside, often with, the qualified nurse professional. It is a role that has been and continues to be performed under a bewildering array of titles: for instance, nursing auxiliary, nursing assistant, assistant nurse, healthcare care assistant, ward assistant, and clinical support worker. As a previous Minster of State for Health, John Denham (Hansard, 1999), noted:

> There is no fixed definition of what an HCA is or does. In the service itself, the term HCA is often used interchangeably with titles used for other staff who undertake similar roles and provide similar support, for example healthcare support workers, nursing auxiliaries and nursing assistants.

These differences in job title are not without significance. They are a testament to the evolution of the role over a considerable period of time, the various titles sometimes being associated with past conceptions of the role and its purpose. Such an accumulation of titles is not, however, without drawbacks. Their continued application to the nurse support role at any given time creates uncertainties about the nature of the role and data on it. For example, staffing data are sometimes broken down by these different titles, although whether or how they reflect differences in tasks performed remains unclear. The book sometimes draws upon these various titles for the nurse support role: they might be appropriate to a particular time or a place. In the main, however, the term 'healthcare assistant' (HCA) is used.

Acknowledging that the HCA role can be found in different healthcare settings—community and tertiary—the book focuses on the role in secondary or acute healthcare. It seeks to provide some context for the HCA role in secondary healthcare by exploring its development across space, that is, in different countries, and time, that is, how it has evolved. Moving forwards to focus on the HCA in Britain, the book unpacks the policy and practitioner objectives underpinning the use of the role, arguing that the viability of these aspirations rests on answers to four basic questions:

1. Are HCAs used as a strategic resource?
2. Who are HCAs?
3. What do they do?
4. How does their role impact on various interested parties:
   - the HCA themselves;
   - the nurses they work with; and
   - the patients they care for?

The core of the book is devoted to addressing these questions. In doing so it draws upon findings from four multi-method hospital case studies in the English National Health Service (NHS). Our research approach allowed us to generate a rich evidence base, which not only comprised qualitative and quantitative material, but also captured the perspectives of different actors with a stake in the role.

The book is divided into ten chapters. The first three provide a backdrop by looking at: the general character and evolution of the HCA role; the policy objectives underpinning the development of the role, which help to frame our research questions; and the research design adopted in pursuing them. The succeeding six chapters present our empirical findings as they relate to the four research questions outlined earlier. The final chapter provides an overview and draws out some lessons for policymakers and practitioners.

The book argues that individuals come to the HCA role with personal characteristics and life histories which distinguish them from qualified nurses, and suggests that they bring distinctive capabilities and qualities to nursing care. The role they perform, in terms of tasks and responsibilities, is highly malleable, assuming varied forms within and between hospital Trusts. The single job title, HCA, hides diverse ways in which the role is shaped and enacted, raising questions about the range of influences on its contours. We reveal that the role is often viewed in extremely positive terms by post holders, nurses, and patients, but also pinpoint some uncertainties, ambiguities, and tensions in the way these stakeholders relate to it. We suggest that the role has the potential to meet policymaker and practitioner objectives, but remain critical of organizational approaches adopted to its use and management. There is scant evidence to indicate that nurse support workers are viewed or used as a strategic resource, casting some doubt upon the capacity for the role to realize its potential. We conclude by suggesting that the role is likely to assume increasing importance as the NHS seeks to cope with new and more intense pressures. The challenges still confronting policymakers and practitioners in developing and managing the HCA role therefore need to be addressed with some urgency.

Chapter 1

Understanding the healthcare assistant role

Introduction

This chapter considers the development of the healthcare assistant (HCA) role in different countries and particularly in Britain. This has value in a number of respects. First, it is a means of more clearly defining the form assumed by the role and how it is positioned in the nursing workforce.

Second, it is an acknowledgement that as policymakers and practitioners address their nursing workforces, in response to new challenges, they are confronted, and, to some extent, constrained, by the path-dependent nature of workforce developments. More specifically, the distribution of nursing tasks and responsibilities across the healthcare workforce, and to the HCA role, is deeply rooted in the evolution of policy and practice over many years. Contemporary HCA roles are the product of a long history, which has shaped what they do, how they are perceived, and how they are managed.

Third, assessing the development of the role provides an opportunity to explore its sensitivity to national culture and institutions. In part this overlaps with the interest in path dependence: the development of the national nursing workforce, and the role of the assistant within it, will be closely tied to the broader evolution of public policy as it relates to provision of health and social care. These national differences also highlight the fact that the structure of national nursing workforces, particularly the distribution of tasks across them, is socially and politically constructed. There is no single, set way of allocating tasks across different occupational groups, so providing scope for countries to look across to one another and consider other possibilities in their approach to work roles. At the same time, such comparisons need to be undertaken with some care. As already implied, national path dependence suggests that the distribution of nursing and related tasks is likely to be deeply embedded in the political economy of healthcare delivery, rendering any simple transfer of practice problematic. It is a warning which equally applies to our review of the evidence on the HCA role in different countries: the embedded nature of the role heavily qualifies the lessons that can be drawn from country-specific research.

This chapter is divided into three substantive parts: the first provides an overview of the development and use of HCAs in a selection of countries; the second sharpens the focus by locating and defining the HCA role in Britain; and the third, looks at the general development of this role, in particular, the factors leading to the heightened importance attached to it in recent years by policymakers and practitioners. However, before moving to these parts, a few conceptual distinctions are made as a starting point for characterizing and analysing HCA roles.

Conceptualizing the healthcare assistant role

It is important initially to unpack the HCA role, distinguishing its different dimensions. This allows us to consider how the role might vary both within and between countries. The first and most basic dimension relates to *who precisely the assistant is assisting*. There are three possibilities:

- The professional;
- The service user;
- The work team or group.

Most obviously, it would appear that the assistant is supporting a professional. Thus, drawing upon assistant roles across the public services, it is striking how they have emerged in harness with a profession: the teaching assistant with the teacher, the community support officer with the police officer, the social work assistant with the social worker, and of course the HCA with the registered nurse. However, working alongside does not necessarily mean that the support workers' primary purpose is to assist the professional. Such a role might equally seek to assist the service user. In education, for example, the teaching assistant is often supporting the special needs pupil rather than the teacher; while in social care, the recently emerged cadre of personal assistants has typically been directly employed by the service user to address their particular needs. Equally the assistant might be supporting the work team or group, becoming a shared resource to be drawn upon as and when required by all team members. Clearly these different forms of assistance—to the professional, to the service user, or to the team—are not mutually exclusively, and might well be closely related. However, the design of the role and/or the way in which stakeholders cognitively engage with it, might display an emphasis toward one rather than the other.

The second dimension relates to the *duties performed* by the assistant. In an acute healthcare context, tasks and responsibilities might broadly be seen to fall into the following categories:

- Auxiliary: routine, low skilled, 'housekeeping' involving little if any direct contact with the patients;

- Caring: semi-skilled and patient centred, in the form of meeting basic care needs;
- Technical: higher-skilled, clinical intervention to assess or deal with patients' conditions;
- Medical: high-skilled, specialist, complex clinical interventions to assess or deal with patients' conditions.

These various types of activity allow for the classification of assistant roles according to the breadth and complexity of the tasks performed. In terms of breadth, the assistant might score 'high'—working across a number of these categories—or 'low'—working within, say, only one. In terms of complexity, the assistant might score 'high'—working in one or both of the last two categories—or 'low'—working in one or both of the first two. This categorization also raises the possibility that in any given country these tasks might be performed by various assistant or support roles.

The third dimension concerns *regulation* of the role. Regulation is designed to control entry into and performance once in the role. This control is mainly a means of ensuring service quality, providing implicit guarantees on the capabilities of the service provider. Such guarantees might, however, be costly, encouraging public policy debate on the value of regulation particularly if the risks associated with the role are low.

Regulation is more or less robust depending on the use and enforcement of the following practices:

- Entry requirements, in the form of training and proven capabilities;
- A Code of Practice, providing guidance on acceptable behaviour and standards;
- Continuing development to ensure that competence is up to date and sustained;
- Registration, providing an accessible and transparent list of capable and approved practitioners;
- Disciplinary procedures dealing with breaches of competence or standards, at the extreme removing the authority for an individual to perform in the role;
- A protected job title, ensuring that only those meeting the listed criteria can use the appropriate designation.

Historically, some occupations have seen labour and/or product market value in regulating themselves, and taken the initiative in setting up their own procedures and mechanisms, an obvious example being traditional craft groups. There has also been a public interest in regulating certain work groups, with policymakers therefore establishing a statutory model of enforcement. Statutory frameworks have, however, varied in terms of the level of prescription and central control. In Britain, the statutory model of regulation has been largely permissive, allowing the professions to adopt a tight form of self-regulation.

More generally, four 'ideal type' models of regulation can be distinguished (Department of Health, 2009a), mainly differentiated by where responsibility lies for establishing and maintaining occupational capabilities and standards:

- *Statutory regulation:* regulation rests with a body comprising experts and possibly representatives from the group in question and is set up by statute, although often operating independently from the state. Such a body will create and service a register, with scope to 'strike-off' an individual who has breached a regulatory requirement.

- *Employer-led regulation:* regulatory responsibility resides with the employer of the workers concerned, and as a result is mainly managed through the individual's contract of employment. In such circumstances, handling serious breaches in regulatory requirements lies in the termination of the employment contract.

- *Occupational licensing:* meeting regulatory requirements rests heavily on the individual worker, who needs a licence to perform in the role. Clearly, an independent licensing authority is still essential to this model, therefore overlapping in part with the first option. Licensing is, however, a less institutionalized approach to statutory regulation, placing great discretion and responsibility on the individual worker to meet the required standards and acquire the appropriate accreditation.

- *(Assured) Voluntary registration:* this model of regulation also places the main onus upon the employee. In placing themselves on a register, practitioners not only indicate their availability for work in a particular role, but signal their acquisition of certain qualifications. In so doing they are providing potential service users and employers with guarantees as to their capabilities. Clearly, the value of such a register is dependent on the criteria set down for registration. An assured system of voluntary registration would be maintained and overseen by an independent body. Inevitably it would, however, be a very 'light-touch' approach: by definition, the lack of compulsions still allows individuals to avoid registration, and makes it difficult for service users and employers to authenticate the status of those who take this course.

The final dimension associated with the assistant role centres on the *ratio of assistants employed* to professionals, and perhaps to other work groups.

In healthcare and some other service areas, this is usually referred to as skill mix. A high ratio of assistants to professionals would be presented as a diluted skill mix, and a lower ratio, a richer skill mix. There has been considerable debate on appropriate skill mix levels in a secondary healthcare setting, the acuity of the patients' conditions, and the size of the ward, often being seen as crucial determinants. A hospital will often have a 'headline' assistant–nurse skill mix of around 40/60 or 30/70. But skill mix will vary by clinical area, naturally being richer in the provision of intensive and critical care, and perhaps more diluted where patient conditions are more stable, for example, in stroke or geriatric wards.

These dimensions of the assistant role, summarized in Figure 1.1, will be drawn upon throughout the book, and in the next section provides the basis for exploring the form assumed by role in countries beyond Britain.

A cross-national comparison of healthcare assistant roles

A cross-national review of the HCA role according to these dimensions highlights important differences, as well as some interesting similarities between countries. Table 1.1 gives a schematic overview from at least two countries in each of the major global regions: Africa, North and South America, Oceania, Asia, and Europe. The data need to be treated with care. They are drawn from various secondary sources, rather than from a single, standard source, with some unevenness, therefore, in terms of the detail and the definitions used. For example, in only a few of the countries is it possible to distinguish HCAs (and nurses) who work in an acute and a community setting. Moreover, these data lack detail on the tasks undertaken by HCAs. Indeed, we know from our research (see Chapter 2) that a single, formal job title hides considerable variation in the shape of the role. The material used in Table 1.1 also lacks the

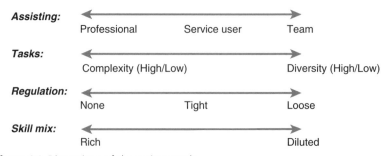

Figure 1.1 Dimensions of the assistant role.

Table 1.1 A cross-national comparison of assistant roles

	Structure of nursing workforce	Task	Regulation	Skill mix
Africa				
Kenya (Dovlo, 2004; Hongoro and McPake, 2004; Munjanja et al., 2005)	Enrolled nurse Care aid instructor Clinical officer/ medical assistant Care assistant	'Nurse aids, medical assistants, clinical officers doing essential medical tasks ... despite professional restrictions' (Hongoro and McPake, 2004: 1453)	Pre-requisites for enrolled/ auxiliary nurses: primary or middle school education	4900 doctors 4300 clinical officers/ assistants medical
South Africa (Hongoro and McPake, 2004; Munjanja et al., 2005; South African Nursing Council, 1991)	Registered nurse Enrolled nurse Nursing auxiliary	Nursing auxiliaries: hands-on patient care including—hygiene, meals, wound care, administration	Nursing auxiliary/enrolled nurse training Requirements: in Nursing Act, 1978 Nursing auxiliary training: pre-technical 10–12 years; basic technical 2 years	Registered nurses: 115,244 Enrolled nurses: 52,370 Nursing auxiliaries: 63,472
North America				
USA (US Bureau of Labor Statistics, 2011)	Registered nurse Licensed practice nurse Nurse assistant also known as nurse aide, nursing assistant, certified nursing assistant	Hands-on patient care including—hygiene, meals, wound care, administration	Nurse assistant Federal training requirement: 75 hours of state approved training and a pass in competency evaluation, which leads to a Certificate 111 needed to practice as a Certified Nursing Assistant. Also Uncertified aides.	Registered nurses: 3,200,200 Licensed practice nurses: 573,600 Nursing aides: 1,469,800

(Cotninued)

Table 1.1 A cross-national comparison of assistant roles (Continued)

	Structure of nursing workforce	Task	Regulation	Skill mix
Canada (Government of Canada, 2011; HRSDC, 2006; Nursing Assistant Canada, 2011)	Registered nurse Licensed practice nurse -Nurse assistant also known as nurse aide, nursing assistant, certified nursing assistant	Hands-on patient care Taking vital signs Record keeping and administration	Nurse aides not nationally regulated Some provinces have preferences, e.g. complete college programme	'Assisting Occupations in Support of health services': 283,335 Registered nurses: 279,399
South America				
Brazil (Gottems et al, 2007; Malvarez and Castrillon, 2005; Ministry of Health, 2006; Neves and Mauro, 2000)	Nurse Technical nurse Nursing auxiliary Aide/nursing attendant	Majority of nursing care provided by nursing auxiliaries	Law 7.498/86, 1986 regulates the practice of nursing auxiliaries Nursing auxiliaries: 1-year nurse training Aides: no specific training	Nurses: 87,100 Technical nurses: 91,935 Nursing auxiliaries: 424, 017 Aides: 57,462
Colombia (Nigenda et al 2010; Pan American Health Organization, 2007)	Licensed nurse Auxiliary nurse	Hands-on patient care	Only basic education required	Licensed nurses: 27,034 Auxiliary nurses: 86,000

Australia and Oceania

Australia (Australian Nursing Federation, 2011)	Registered nurse Enrolled nurse Assistants in nursing	Hands-on patient care	Assistants in nursing have no regulation or consistent educational preparation	Registered nurses: 271,949 (incl. public private) Acute setting 132,744 public/ 39,512 private Enrolled nurses: 62,079 Assistants in nursing: 73,000
New Zealand (Nursing Council of New Zealand, 2010)	Registered nurse Enrolled nurse Healthcare assistant	Hands-on patient care. HCA specializations, e.g. care of the elderly	No regulation or consistent educational preparation	Registered nurses: 43,826 (18,415 acute) Enrolled nurses/ HCAs: 3238 (acute 843)

Asia

Japan (LPN Duties, 2011; Ministry of Health, Labour and Welfare, 2009; Sawada, 1997; Tierney and Tierney, 1994)	Nurse License practice nurse Assistant nurse	Hands-on patient care; vital signs; record keeping	Assistant nurses are licensed; license issued after completing two years of training	Nurses: 660,142 (FTE) Assistant nurses: 66,546
China (Kalisch and Liu, 2009; Xu et al, 2000)	Registered nurse Nurse assistant	Most care provide by the patient's family, who also directly employ the nursing assistant	Unclear	Unclear

(Cotinued)

Table 1.1 A cross-national comparison of assistant roles (Continued)

	Structure of nursing workforce	Task	Regulation	Skill mix
Europe				
Germany (European Commission, 2000; Statistisches Bundesamt, 2010)	First level nurses: General nurse Paediatric nurse Geriatric nurse Second level: Assistants nurse	Hands-on patient care; vital signs; record keeping	Assistants (and nurses) need a permit to practise Responsibility for permit at regional level 1-year course based in school of nursing	Assistant nurses: 558,000
Spain (Camano-Puig, 2005; Gonzalez and Barber, 2009)	Registered nurse Nursing assistant	'Activities complementing those of the registered nurse' (Camano-Puig, 2005: 59)	Unregulated	Nurses: 130,345 Nursing assistants: 106,843
Sweden (Daly and Szebehely, 2011; Hasson and Arnetz, 2008; Simoens et al, 2005)	Registered nurse Licensed practice nurse Nursing assistant	Hands-on care; administration of some medication	Unregulated	Assistant nurses: 163,200 (represents 58% of the nursing workforce)

depth to explore precisely who the assistant is supporting: the first substantive column, therefore, sets out the structure of the nursing workforce in the respective countries. Moreover the data presented provide a snapshot of assistant roles in the respective countries, limiting the scope to assess change.

Accepting these limitations, it is still possible to highlight a number of interesting patterns in the use and nature of the HCA role in different countries. More specifically, the following points emerge from Table 1.1:

• The registered nurse is often supported by a number of nurse assistant roles. This is not only reflected in the variety of job titles used for the nurse support role within the same country, which may or may not reflect differences in function, but more formally in various levels of the assistant role. The most common pattern is for a three-tier nursing workforce structure, with a middle nurse support tier falling between the registered nurse and the non-qualified assistant, and requiring post holders to acquire some formal level of accredited training. This middle tier is referred to as: the enrolled nurse (South Africa, Australia, New Zealand); the licensed practice nurse (USA, Canada, Japan, Sweden), or nurse auxiliary (Brazil). At the same time, there are other nursing workforces with a simpler bifurcated structure, the registered nurse working alongside a single assistant role (Columbia, China, Spain).

• There are difficulties in discerning precisely who the assistant is assisting. However, there are instances, in particular China, and to a lesser extent Spain, where the family is responsible for much of the patient care in an acute setting. In such cases, nurse support workers are employed by the family and provide direct assistance to the patient rather than the nurse professional.

• In the main, tasks performed by HCAs centre on 'hands-on' patient care, that is, meeting basic patient needs through tasks such as feeding, bed making, and washing. It is noteworthy that in some countries assistants routinely appear to undertake low-level technical tasks such as monitoring vital signs (Canada, Japan, and Germany). There are isolated instances where the assistant role is formally extended to high-level technical tasks such as administering medication (Sweden), and less formally where the shortages of registered nurses encourage assistants to take on such tasks (Kenya).

• Table 1.1 reveals a variety of regulatory models for assistant roles. Middle tier, enrolled nurse roles are typically founded on mandatory pre-entry training. However, the assistant role is often unregulated, with no entry requirements or means of ensuring the maintenance of capabilities and standards (Canada, Brazil, Colombia, Australia, New Zealand, Spain, and Sweden). There are some instances where the role is more formally regulated. In South Africa, for example, this takes the form of a pre-entry, two-year period of training. In Germany, Japan, and the USA regulation is founded upon a licensing model, assistants needing a certificate to practise. This model is most robustly applied in Japan and Germany where assistant nurses can only practise with a licence: there appears to be no unregulated assistant roles in these two countries. In the USA, non-licensed nurse aides can be employed, performing a narrower and less technical range of tasks than those with a licence.

• As suggested, it is difficult to make an accurate assessment of skill mix, particularly in an acute care setting, on the basis of these data. However, in crude terms, a number of different patterns can be discerned. A 2:1 ratio between qualified/registered nurses and non-qualified/non-registered assistants (the latter including enrolled nurses) might be viewed as a 'middling' skill mix: after all, given that nurses are the most formally qualified group within the nursing workforce, a 2:1 ratio with assistants would seem to fall between a rich and diluted skill mix. Such a 2:1 skill mix was found in a number of countries (USA, Australia, and Sweden). Another group of countries have a more diluted skill mix, the ratio approaching 50/50 split (South Africa, Canada, and Spain). These sit alongside others with a heavily diluted skill mix: that is, where the number of assistants far exceeded nurses. This appeared to be the pattern in South American countries (Brazil and Colombia). There was a further group of countries with a rich skill mix. In such cases there were three or four times as many nurses to assistants (Japan and New Zealand).

In summary, it is clear that the form assumed by the assistant role varies between countries across our four dimensions. There are some regionally-based patterns. For example, the structure of the nursing workforce in the USA and Canada, as well as in Australia and New Zealand, is very similar. We have also seen that in both the South American countries included in the analysis— Brazil and Columbia—skill mix remained highly diluted. However, the differences revealed by our analysis suggest patterns which cut across global region. The positioning of the assistant role within the nursing workforce assumed two forms: as the only nurse support role, or sitting beneath a more formalized, middle-tier, enrolled nurse. The tasks performed by the assistant role essentially focused on hands-on direct care, but there were instances where the role had routinely been extended to take on low-level, and even higher-level, technical tasks. In many countries, regulation of the assistant role was absent. There were, however, instances where formal, pre-entry training was required, while some countries were using a licensing model, albeit differing in how tightly entry was controlled into the assistant role. The most striking differences related to skill mix. Although data on workforce numbers by role need to be treated with the most care, it was clear that countries ranged from those with a highly diluted to those with a highly enriched nursing workforce.

This cross-country comparison suggests different trajectories for the development of the assistant role. Certainly it indicates the assistant role's sensitivity to broader social and political factors, not least related to the development of national healthcare systems, and perhaps the scope for some public policy discretion in, or choice on, the shaping of the nursing workforce. It also provides a context and a benchmark for exploring the HCA role in Britain, and particularly England. This exploration begins in the next section with an attempt to define the HCA, before we move on to consider how the role has developed in recent years.

Locating support roles in Britain

Definitions and numbers

As a generic role, the support worker can be found in a range of health and social care sector settings in Britain. In a broad definition of the role, Saks and Allsop (2007) view support workers as those:

> … who provide face to face care or support of a personal or confidential nature to service users in a clinical or therapeutic setting, community facilities or domiciliary context, but who do not hold a qualification accredited by a professional association and are not formally regulated by a statutory body.

This is a definition which leads the authors to suggest that around one million such workers can be found across Britain, a considerably higher number than any registered group of health or social care workers.

In a more refined definition, relating to staff specifically employed in the NHS, the Scottish Executive defines the 'Heath Care Support Worker' role as (NMC, 2006):

> Those who provide a direct service – that is they have direct influence/effect on patient care/treatment/relationships – to patients and members of the public … This would include those in support roles to healthcare professions (such as care assistants) and those who provide ancillary services (such as porters and mortuary attendants).

Clearly this is a definition broad enough to capture ancillary staff such as porters and cleaners, as well as those more directly assisting the nurse and other healthcare professionals. Using such a definition, the number of support workers in the NHS in England is best calculated by drawing upon those workers officially classified as 'supporting clinical staff' (The Health and Social Care

Information Centre, 2011), a group subdivided into those providing support to: doctors and nurses; scientific, therapeutic, and technical staff; and ambulance staff. In 2010, the full-time equivalent (FTE) number of staff across these subcategories stood at 307,000, a 45 per cent rise from the 211,000 employed in 1995.

The Nursing and Midwifery Council (NMC) (NMC, 2006), distinguishing HCAs as a subset of the 'healthcare support workers', explicitly draws upon the definition developed by the Scottish Executive, but tightens it up:

> Those who provide a direct service – that is they have a direct influence/effect on care/treatment to patients and members of the public and are supervised by and/or undertake healthcare duties delegated to them by NMC registrants.

Such a tightening leads to a more refined definition, with ancillary staff now excluded, and HCAs more sharply defined as a discrete group directly supervised by the registered nurse. Under this definition HCAs would fall under the official category of 'supporting doctors and nurses'. This category does not completely overlap with the HCA role, comprising other groups of staff such as administrative workers. But considering those workers who fall under this heading and within the NMC definition, there has been a 26 per cent rise in HCAs over the last ten years: the FTE numbers increasing from around 93,000 in 1995 to some 117,000 in 2010.

This modest rise is indicated in Figure 1.2. The material presented in this figure draws upon Department of Health data, which continues to be collected on the basis of a distinction between 'healthcare assistant' and 'nurse auxiliary/assistant' roles. How trusts define workers for these purposes and whether these titles reflect 'real' differences in nurse support roles within and between Trusts remains unclear. When data on nurse support numbers are set alongside changes in the numbers of registered nurses over the same period, four phases in staffing emerge which might speculatively be related to broader public policy developments:

- *1995–2000:* the first phase is the back-end of the Conservative period of government and the start of the New Labour period—the number of registered nurses remained relatively stable, while nurse support workers increased. This was a time when the Conservative's local HCA grade was perhaps taking-off. NHS expenditure also remained tight, New Labour, for example, initially committing itself to Conservative expenditure plans, possibly encouraging the use of the 'cheaper' nurse support worker option.

- *2001–2005:* there followed a phase characterized by a steep rise in nurse numbers, with those in nurse support roles increasing on a much more modest scale. This was a time when New Labour investment in the NHS

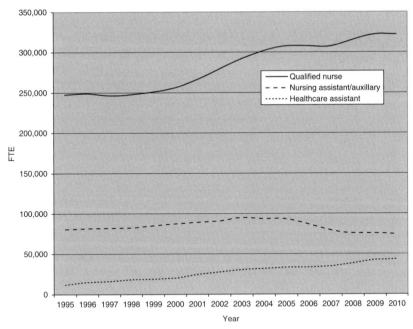

Figure 1.2 NHS full-time equivalent staff (1995–2010). Source: The Information Centre for Health and Social Care, Non-Medical Workforce Census. Copyright © 2011, Re-used with the permission of The Health and Social Care Information Centre. All rights reserved.

was taking-off and the NHS Plan, 2000, established targets for the recruitment of registered nurses. Indeed the NHS Plan set a target of 20,000 additional nurses by 2004, a target in practice met by 2002.

• *2005–2008:* a third phase is marked by a continued if slightly reduced rate of growth in registered nurses and a levelling off in nurse support numbers—the rise in 'healthcare assistants' is countered by a fall in 'nurse assistants/auxiliaries', presumably indicative of the growing use of the latter job title and the expense of the former ones.

• *2008–2010:* a final phase sees a slight downturn in registered nurse numbers, as those in HCA posts gently rise.

These trends find a further expression in patterns of skill mix over these years, as set out in Figure 1.3. The phases in this figure broadly map on to those identified in Figure 1.2: a sharp dilution of skill mix until 2000 as nurse numbers remain stable while nurse support workers increase; a skill mix plateau, before a sharp move to skill mix enrichment down to 2008, when again there is a flattening out.

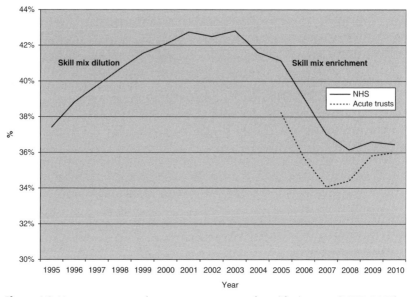

Figure 1.3 Nurse support workers as a percentage of qualified nurses (1995–2010). Source: The Information Centre for Health and Social Care, Non-Medical Workforce Census. Copyright © 2011, Re-used with the permission of The Health and Social Care Information Centre. All rights reserved.

With these HCAs spread across the health service, the numbers in a secondary or acute healthcare setting still need to be established. This is not a straightforward task: a breakdown of staff groups by healthcare setting is only provided as far back as 2005. Over the period 2005–2010 secondary healthcare remained the main setting for the employment of HCAs, but it is noteworthy that the numbers (FTE) remained stable at 60,000 over this period, suggesting some caution in proclaiming the inexorable rise of the HCA. Moreover, this was a time when the number of qualified nurses in this subsector increased from 158,000 to 167,000, a 5.7 per cent increase. As can be seen again from Figure 1.3, this is reflected in a marked enrichment of the skill mix over the 2005–2008 period, mirroring the trend in the wider NHS. Similarly there follows a flattening of skill mix between 2008–2010, with not far short of three nurses to every HCA in secondary healthcare.

The nature of the role and its regulation

The various definitions of the support worker provide some clue as to the nature of the HCA role. They suggest that any characterization can be related to intrinsic functionality—what post holders actually do—and to the way in which the role is managed. In terms of functionality, the notion of a support role returns us to our question about whom or what is actually being supported. The Saks and Allsop definition places considerable emphasis on service user support, as does the Scottish Executive definition, with the weight given to the role's 'direct influence or effect on patient care'. The NMC definition brings to the fore the HCA's relationship with the care professional. It stresses the HCA's role alongside and possibly in support of the nurse, implicit in the assumption that the latter delegates to the former. This closeness to the professional is crucial in affecting the possible contours of the HCA role: it remains an empirical question as to whether and in what ways the HCA supports the nurse, and whether they deliver hands-on care, but it is this potential to work in harness with the nurse and to provide such care which distinguishes the HCA from those in ancillary health support roles such as porters and cleaners.

In defining support roles, Saks and Allsop stress the absence of statutory regulation and the scope to undertake the role without any accredited qualification. As we have seen in the cross-national comparison, this is not intrinsic to the role but rather a (default) public policy choice. HCAs in England *de facto* remain unregulated. For much of the post-1945 period there was a state enrolled nurse position, but following a reorganization of nurse training in the mid-1990s under Project 2000, the position was withdrawn, leaving in place a nursing workforce with a simple twofold structure: registered and unregistered.

There has, however, been much debate over whether and how support roles in health should be regulated. Indeed, the intensity of such debates has increased in recent years as a number of high-profile cases have related care failures, in part, to skill mix issues. A Healthcare Commission inquiry (2007: 64) into some 90 deaths between April 2004 and September 2006 at Maidstone and Tunbridge Wells NHS Trust 'definitely or probably' related to an outbreak of *Clostridium difficile*, noted that a high proportion of medical and surgical wards (80%), 'were staffed below the national average for the percentage of qualified nurses.' Similarly, an inquiry into the Mid Staffordshire NHS Foundation Trust (Francis, 2010), recording 400 more deaths than expected between 2005–2008, drew attention to a decision to dilute skill mix from 60:40 to 40:60 on the medical wards, while also recounting a range of ('unsatisfactory') patient care experiences involving HCAs.

Notwithstanding these cases, the path towards any form of HCA regulation has proved a long and tortuous one, revealing tensions amongst stakeholders and particularly dilemmas for government policymakers. The New Labour government unambiguously presented the goal of regulation as a patient safety issue, but set out criteria for the introduction of statutory regulation, including the need for it to be proportionate, transparent, and consistent. As far back as 2000, the English NHS Plan registered a commitment to consider proposals for the effective regulation of support workers (Department of Health, 2006a). A consultation exercise on the issue suggested 'a strong overall case for extending regulation to at least some support workers' (p. 33). UNISON and the Royal College of Nurses (RCN) have both been vociferous in their support of HCA regulation, albeit through different regulatory bodies, the former favouring the Health Professions Council and the latter the NMC. However, the New Labour government (Department of Health, 2007a) consistently deferred any decision to the completion of a pilot project in Scotland on HCA regulation, overseen by a four-country steering group.

The Scottish pilot tested a model of employer-led regulation in three of its NHS boards and in one independent hospital during 2007–2008. The model comprised: a set of induction standards for healthcare support workers (HSW); Codes of Practice for HSWs and employers; and a centrally-held list of those who met the standards. In response to this pilot, the induction standards and the Codes of Practice were implemented in the Scottish NHS, from 31 December 2010. This lead was followed by Wales, which also introduced Codes of Practice for HSWs and for NHS employers in the country.

However, despite a continued clamour for the regulation of HCAs in England, not least expressed by the head of the NMC who labelled the unregistered healthcare workforce on hospital wards as a 'ghastly national disaster' waiting to happen (Nursing Times, 2011), there has been little appetite to move forward with a robust approach. The Working Group on Extending Professional and Occupational Regulation (Department of Health, 2009a: 35) explicitly ruled out full-blown statutory regulation for HCAs, suggesting a 'lighter touch' employer-led or licensing approach. Indeed, this has arguably been watered down even further by the Conservative-led coalition whose preferred solution is a system of assured voluntary registration to be overseen by the Council for Healthcare Regulatory Excellence (Department of Health, 2011)

In summary, this section has located the HCA as a role which engages directly with the patient and works alongside, often under, the direction of the registered nurse. In Britain, this nurse support activity has remained relatively undifferentiated in occupational terms, and particularly since the demise of the state enrolled nurse. It has also remained an unregulated part of the nursing workforce, in the face of increasingly intense and ongoing debate over the need for and viability of such regulation. As a means of developing a fuller appreciation of the current state and status of the HCA, the next section looks in greater detail at the evolution of the role.

Evolution of the role

Historical context

The proliferation of assistants in various parts of the public services over recent years belies important differences in the development in these roles. In primary and secondary education, the teaching assistant had some grounding in the traditional school workforce, combining the established special needs assistant and the classroom helper roles. However, the teaching assistant was tightly tied to the New Labour modernization project, illustrated by a 190 per cent growth in the number of teaching assistants between 1997–2007, from 61,000 to 177,000, as the number of teachers rose by 11 per cent, from 399,000 to 444,000 (Bach and Kessler, 2011: 105). The community support officer (CSO) in the police force was even more closely aligned to this phase of public service reform, being introduced to undertake neighbourhood liaison activities, so releasing warranted police officers to concentrate on dealing with more serious criminal activities. The scale of the CSO workforce was relatively modest, at around 17,000 by 2009 but given that the role was introduced for the first time in 2002, this constitutes a noteworthy figure.

In contrast, the HCA role has been much more deeply embedded in the traditional healthcare workforce. This section will argue that various pressures have certainly heightened the importance of the HCA role and opened-up a new, broader space for its performance. However, it will also become apparent that the contemporary development of the HCA still bears the hallmarks of its history.

A nurse support role has been a longstanding feature of the nursing workforce, dating back to the beginnings of modern nursing. Stokes and Warden (2004) highlight the presence of nurses' aides during the Crimean War, 1854–1856, and track the development of the role over the following century and a half. This development has been punctuated by a number of key events. Nursing was established as a registered profession under the Health Care Act, 1919. However, this registration failed to ensure complete closure for 'qualified' nurses, continuing to allow non-registered workers as part of the nursing workforce. In 1955 the 'nursing auxiliary' role was given formal recognition in the healthcare setting, but coexisted alongside a qualified assistant nurse. The two-year assistant nurse qualification did not allow registration as nurses, but did lead to inclusion on a Roll of Nurses, and in 1961 to the designation State Enrolled Nurses (SEN) (Webb, 2000).

Tracing the development of the non-qualified nursing auxiliary in the 20 or 30 years following its formal recognition in 1955 is far from straightforward, not least given the paucity of evidence on the nature of the role. Certainly there are data to suggest that numbers in the role grew rapidly in the 1960s and 1970s. In 1965 there were almost 46,000 nursing auxiliaries in a hospital setting. By 1975 this number had almost doubled to 77,000. The increased numbers of enrolled nurses over this same period was also striking: they doubled from 22,300 to 44,500. Indeed, the growth of both groups of workers is particularly noteworthy alongside the more modest growth of registered nurses in hospitals over this time, with an increase from 65,700 to 83,000 (Snee, 1978).

As implied, the shape and nature of the nurse auxiliary role at this time remains much more elusive. The Briggs report (Briggs, 1972) reviewing the nurse role and nurse training in the early 1970s, makes few references to the nurse auxiliary. Certainly, the report acknowledges a nurse support role within the ward team (pp. 199–200), proposing a change in job title from 'auxiliary' to 'nursing aide'. There was, however, little attempt to explore the substance of the role, or whether a change of title was designed to reflect a change of function or purpose. The report limited its comments on such workers to the somewhat vague suggestion that 'there should be maximum use of aides both in the hospital and the community and their work should be related very directly to the work of other members of nursing or midwifery teams' (p. 40). Indeed, while the Briggs report moves on to explore relations at the 'borderline' between nurses and doctors, nurses and allied health professionals, nurses and groups outside the NHS, and nurses and volunteers, it completely fails to consider the nurse–auxiliary/aide borderline. This is in contrast to Allen's (2001) study of the nurse role some 30 years later which similarly took a 'borders' approach, the nurse–support worker border being the first it considered.

Fragmentary evidence suggests that the nurse auxiliary role, often revolved around 'dirty work'—emptying commodes and cleaning out sluices. As Johnson (1978) with a touch of irony notes in describing the role, 'The auxiliary [is] delegated such noble tasks as walking the elderly patient to the lavatory or changing the sheets of the incontinent' (p. 112). This impression is reinforced by the Briggs report, which almost inadvertently hints at the low level nature of the tasks traditionally performed by auxiliaries. In a survey of around 1600 nursing auxiliaries, carried out for the report, exactly half had neither received an induction or 'any later training'. With only 25 per cent of the remaining half receiving 'any later training' (the other quarter receiving just induction), it is clear that only a small proportion of auxiliaries appeared equipped to extend their role much beyond basic support tasks.

From the mid-1980s, however, a series of related developments propelled the nurse support worker to the fore in terms of public policy and practice, in the process creating much greater visibility for the role and challenging its shadowy status.

Project 2000

The first of these developments was a reorganization of nurse work and training. It was an initiative founded upon a report written in 1986 by the United Kingdom Central Council (UKCC) for Nursing, Midwifery and Health Visiting entitled *Project 2000: A New Preparation for Practice*. The key recommendations were implemented in 13 demonstration districts in 1989, before being rolled-out across the country (Maben and Macleod Clark, 1998).

Ostensibly Project 2000 centred on a new approach to nurse training, with direct implications for the role of the nurse support worker. This new approach to registered nurse training saw a shift from an apprentice, 'shopfloor' model of training, firmly rooted in hospital schools of nursing, to one based on formal theory and 'classroom' learning in a university or college setting. This change reduced the opportunity for registered nurses to use student nurses as a support, leaving the non-qualified nurse worker as the main source of help. Thus student nurses became largely supernumerary in practice areas, making a rostered contribution to patient care only in the latter stages of their course (Philpin, 1999). Moreover, the government only provided enough funds for half of the new student nurses to be replaced on the wards when they stepped out of practice to study, encouraging the search for cheaper skill mix options, and a further reliance on the nurse support worker.

Indeed such an option was encouraged with the government's introduction of a so-called 'healthcare assistant' role explicitly seen as the replacement for this student nurse support. Introduced as part of the NHS and Community Care Act, 1990, the HCA was established alongside the national Whitley 'nursing auxiliary' grade. It was made available to newly created hospital Trusts as a local grade to be shaped and rewarded as they saw fit.

The change to nurse training prompted by Project 2000 was, however, founded upon a much more radical restructuring of the nursing workforce. This revolved around what the UKCC report labelled 'a practitioner-centred division of labour', which saw the removal of the SEN role. Reflecting different membership interests, the deletion of the SEN had been urged by the RCN but vehemently opposed by other unions, at the time the COHSE and NUPE (subsequently combining with NALGO to form UNISON). In backing the former approach, the UKCC pointed to the frustrations associated with an SEN role, 'caught in the middle' or 'falling between stools'. The UKCC report suggested that SENs were misused 'being treated as one level at one moment, another the next', and abused 'being mistreated as inferior to the first level and lacking knowledge and judgment' (UKCC, 1986: 39). The phasing out of the SEN left the UKCC with a workforce essentially comprising the registered nurse and what they called the aide, with residual scope for the development of a specialist nurse practitioner stream.

The UKCC report also suggested a name change from auxiliary to aide. In contrast to the passing mention of the nurse support role in the Briggs report, the UKCC report recognized the need to elaborate on the nature of this role, not least given its call for a single nurse support tier. Nonetheless, the aide was still presented almost grudgingly by the UKCC, which noted that 'In an ideal world, most would wish to see registered practitioners giving all the care needed'. The report continued: 'It was always clear, however, that in the real world the new practitioner could not practice alone' (pp. 42–3). As implied by this statement, the aide was to be the registered nurses' helper, the UKCC making it clear that the registered nurse was to remain responsible and accountable for the care given, and in a position to monitor its delivery. The UKCC Project 2000 report also called for a formal period of formal induction and preparation for the aide, at around three months.

The UKCC Project 2000 changes in nurse training and the deletion of the SEN grade as suggested were implemented, although some of the more detailed suggestions were 'left on the shelf'. The 'aide' job title was crowded out by the myriad of existing titles—nurse auxiliary, nurse assistant—and overtaken by new ones—healthcare assistant and, under Agenda for Change, clinical support worker. More significantly, the call for a standard preparation for those in the nurse support role gave way to a much more formal process of accreditation, which linked post holder capabilities to NVQ (National Vocation Qualification) levels 2 and 3, albeit on a discretionary basis and without these qualifications becoming formal entry requirements to the role.

Indeed, this accreditation introduced some differentiation in to the nurse support role and its post holders. While the passing of the SEN role removed a qualified layer of nurse support, a degree of formal hierarchy remained in the non-qualified nurse support workforce. This was linked to the size and complexity of different roles and reflected in various ways. In the early 2000s, a NHS Career Framework was developed which distinguished three main levels for unregistered practitioners: support workers at level 2, senior healthcare assistants at level 3, and assistant or associate practitioners at level 4. At the same time the NHS Modernization Agency's Changing Workforce programme was using this framework to encourage and pilot new support roles. These were taken up by various regions, the North West (Selfe et al., 2008) in particular, seeking to develop assistant practitioner roles at career level 4.

The Whitely pay and grading structure continued to acknowledge some differentiation, with nurse support roles sitting in one of two grades: A or B. Indeed, this differentiation was transposed onto Bands 2 and 3 of the Agenda for Change (AfC), 2004, pay and grading structure, with a Band 4 mapping onto the assistant practitioner level. The Band 2 role spans points 1–8 of the AfC pay spine, giving a range of £13,903–17,003, while Band 3 covers points 6–13 with a range between £15,860 and £18,827 (at 1 April 2011 rates) and the Band 4 bridges 11–17 with a range between £18,402 and £21,625. Registered nurse pay begins at Band 5 and spinal point 16 with a salary of £21,176.

The nurse profession

As Project 2000 was elevating the HCA to the main source of support for the registered nurse, a second set of equally powerful forces was pushing the registered nurses away from the direct provision of patient care: in effect, a broader space was opening up within which the HCA could perform. These forces were partly associated with the broader nurse professionalization project (Doherty, 2007), as registered nurses attempted to move up the clinical ladder by taking on and deepening their technical skills. They were also linked to the broader direction of public policy travel, as governments and Trusts sought to develop the nurse role along these lines. The Department of Health noted in *Modernising Nursing Careers: Setting the Direction* (Department of Health, 2006b: 19):

> Nursing careers in the future will be shaped by the needs of patient and clients. They will encompass the wide range of new and advanced roles, clarify contribution of specialist and generalists roles and show how they fit with the wider workforce.

These aspirations were given form by the emergence of advanced and specialist nurse roles, captured by the generic titles 'advanced nurse practitioner' and 'clinical nurse specialist'. These role types had very different implications for nurse practice, but in general they fragmented the nurse profession, taking it away from holistic care provision.

The scope for the nurse profession to push in this direction, supported by policymakers, was tied to a number of pressing needs encouraging a reorganization and recalibration of clinical tasks. Indeed the strengths of these pressures might be seen in the development of similar roles in countries such as the US, Canada, France, and Finland (Delamaire and Lafortune, 2010), where an OECD report suggested they were:

• a response to shortages in doctors;
• a means of pursuing of higher quality and lower cost healthcare; and
• a way of improving career opportunities for nurses.

Such pressures have had some influence in Britain, while taking a more refined form. There were moves toward new models of care provisions often based upon multiprofessional teams and encouraging the development of new nurse roles. There were also certain skill shortages promoting nurses to take on more technical tasks (Brown and Jones, 2011). Most striking, however, were pressures associated with the European Working Time Directive, enacted in 1998 and taking effect on junior doctors' hours in the NHS in August 2009. It necessitated a reduction in the working week to 48 hours, encouraging, in turn, the delegation of some junior doctors' tasks to nurses, such as taking bloods and cannulation. As Professor Sir John Temple (2010) noted in reviewing the impact of the directive on the quality of junior doctor training:

> There must be a national strategy with clarity on the service responsibilities and cost efficiencies for the development of roles such as physician assistants, specialist nurses, advanced nurse practitioners and surgical care assistants, as these professionals can reduce unnecessary demands on junior trainees.

This delegation of junior doctor tasks to the nurse had a knock-on effect to the HCA role. As the government consultation paper on regulation noted (Department of Health, 2004: 5):

> Unregulated staff, such as healthcare assistants and other support staff are extending their skills so that they can undertake work previously done by registered professionals in order to meet patient needs. This is particularly necessary as nurses and allied health professionals take on extended roles to help employers to meet the European Working Time Directive for doctors.

Mapping the incidence and nature of these new, more specialist nurse roles is far from straightforward. They often emerged opportunistically and organically, giving rise to some public policy concern about their regulation (Brown and Jones, 2011). However, a RCN study (2005) of over 700 nurses performing such roles confirmed their recent growth: it found that most had been introduced in the last four years, 60 per cent of respondents being the first to fill them.

These developments in the nature of the registered nurse workforce sat alongside broader changes related to the modernization of the NHS over recent years, similarly challenging the nurses' presence at the bedside. In general, moves towards an audit- and targets-based performance management culture in the NHS had an important effect on work organization and the nature of the nurse role. In part, this culture placed an increasing emphasis on administration, taking up a growing part of the nurse's working day. An RCN survey of three West Midland Trusts in 2005 revealed that nurses were spending as much as 40 per cent of their time on such work, leading to

RCN General Secretary at the time, Beverley Malone, to note (The Observer, 2005) that:

> The administrative burden is keeping them [nurses] from doing the things that need to be done, whether it's tackling patient safety or infection control or talking to patients. It seems like it's taking up an incredible amount of their time. There are more clerical tasks, more documentation, and targets to meet.

It was a finding confirmed in a later RCN survey in 2008, which suggested that nationally, nurses spent more than a million hours a week on paperwork, with 85 per cent of the 1700 surveyed nurses indicating that more help with such paperwork would allow them to spend more time caring for patients. As the RCN General Secretary, at this time Peter Carter (RCN, 2008), stressed, 'Nurses are clearly feeling the burden of non essential paperwork and the danger is that this is undermining their ability to care for patients and support relatives'.

Nurses were not solely diverted from the bedside by paperwork. In addition, access targets encouraged a focus on a faster, more efficient throughput of patients, with a concomitant requirement on nurses to deal with the procedural complexities surrounding admission and discharge. Regular ward audits of work practices, also associated with the achievement of targets, represented a further 'drain' on the nurses' time.

It remains an empirical question as to how far the registered nurse role has changed in response to the pressures associated with Project 2000 and the development of the nurse profession. In recent years, however, increasing attention has been drawn to the impact of these changes on nurse and HCA roles, and, in turn, to the possible consequences for patient care. In a commentary exploring these issues, senior lecturer in nursing at London South Bank University, Suzanne Fullbrook (2004), suggestively entitled her piece: 'Changing roles and titles: HCAs now deliver the care'. Fullbrook appeared to be in little doubt about this trend, not even framing this title as a question. More prosaically the NMC (2006) has noted:

> There are now significant changes in the way that services are delivered to patients. In particular following the General Medical Services contract and the European Working Time Directive, nurses and midwives and specialist community public health nurses are undertaking treatment and care that was once the domain of other healthcare professionals, notably doctors. Consequently this has led to non-registered staff members delivering some aspects of care previously only undertaken by nurses.

As the government has recently stressed (Department of Health, 2004):

> Unregulated staff, such as healthcare assistants and other support staff are extending their skills so that they can undertake work previously done by registered professionals in order to meet patient needs.

Summary

Found under various job titles, it is now clear that our focus remains a HCA role integral to the nursing workforce in secondary healthcare, typically working alongside the qualified or registered nurse and directly engaging with patient care. This chapter has sought to unpack different dimensions of this role:

- Locus of support: the nurse, the patient and or the team;
- Nature and range of tasks performed: breadth and complexity;
- Degree and nature of regulation: tight or loose;
- Skill mix, the ratio of support to qualified workers: diluted or rich.

   A review of various countries has revealed differences along these dimensions, suggesting the role's sensitivity to broader, path-dependent national institutions of healthcare delivery. Nonetheless, there were patterns in the use and development of the HCA role, in turn, implying constrained national 'choices'. It was clear that the HCA role:

- Often works under another, more 'qualified' nurse support role, sometimes referred to as the enrolled nurse;
- Is typically confined to the provision of basic patient care, but can extend to more technical tasks;
- Is quite commonly an unregulated role, although some countries have sought to license post holders or impose pre-entry training requirements.

   In Britain, the contemporary status of the HCA role saw it as the only direct support for the registered nurse. There has been much recent debate about regulation, with employer-led models of regulation recently emerging in Scotland and Wales. However, in England this issue remains largely unresolved, the likely outcome being a loose form of regulation, based on an assured voluntary register. Certainly there has only been a modest change in the numbers of HCAs over recent years, in contrast to the explosion of assistants in other parts of the public services, and suggesting perhaps that the HCA role had not been as closely aligned with New Labour's public services 'modernization project'.

   These staffing trends, however, belie the growing importance of a nurse support role, deeply embedded in the British nursing workforce, and for many years working alongside the state enrolled nurse. Project 2000, in particular, elevated the HCA to the main source of nurse support as changes in nurse training removed the student nurse to the 'classroom' from the ward, and as the SEN was phased out. This development has been accompanied by the

opening up of a broader space for the performance of the HCA role as registered nurses, seeking to deepen their specialist skills or diverted to administrative work, increasingly appear to have withdrawn from the bedside. Emerging
as the principal ward-based role working alongside the registered nurse, and
functioning in a broader space, the HCA role has attracted increasing attention
from policymakers.

Chapter 2

Healthcare assistants: policy objectives and evidence base

The modern HCA role: policy objectives

The importance of the HCA role to the delivery of healthcare services in the context of the developments outlined in the last chapter has increasingly been recognized by policymakers. In his report for the government on the future of the NHS, Sir Derek Wanless (2002) noted that, 'alongside support for an extension of nurse-led services, there was general agreement that the next twenty years will see an extended role for healthcare assistants'. More recently, the importance of the HCA has been re-asserted, with the NHS Next Stage Review (Department of Health, 2009b) noting that:

> Key to delivering this overall programme are clinical support roles, for example, healthcare assistants. We will work with partners and the profession to ensure that employees in these types of roles are appropriately trained.

Despite the growing importance of the HCA, there have been signs of caution towards the role on the part of policymakers. When the Secretary of State for Health noted in 2008 that, 'Our *nurses* do a brilliant job, often delivering very intimate care' [emphasis added], the HCA contribution appears to have been overlooked, a particularly glaring omission given the increasing the bedside presence of these workers. Indeed, the NHS Plan for England made no specific mention of HCAs at all (Buchan and Seccombe, 2002), and this reluctance to acknowledge their role was noted by Warrington North MP Helen Jones (Hansard, 1999) when she raised the issue in the House of Commons:

> Part of that modernisation [of the NHS] is our commitment to supporting and valuing our staff. In that context, we hear much about doctors and nurses ... however other members of staff are also an important part of the healthcare team; without them our National Health Service could not function. These include the category known as healthcare assistants, or in some Trusts, support workers.

This public policy ambiguity towards HCAs might be seen as related to ongoing and emergent tensions in how the role is perceived. In broad terms, two sets of public policy objectives can be distinguished as underpinning the use of the role. The first views the HCA role in terms of its flexibility and cost efficiency: HCAs are a readily acquired, relatively low-cost resource. The second sees them as more explicitly contributing to the care quality agenda: they might be used in a new and innovative ways to improve the patient experience. Clearly, these sets of objectives are not mutually exclusive, and public policymakers and practitioners would claim a concern both with cost and effectiveness in their use of HCAs.

There are, however, inevitably potential tensions, between cost and effectiveness. As implied in Chapter 1, these tensions have been particularly apparent in heated debates over the regulation of the HCA. In the face of a nurse profession consensus on the need for such regulation as a means of preserving and ensuring care quality, governments of different party political complexions have displayed a remarkably consistent approach, cautioning against a regulatory approach which might impose high costs and rigidities. In rejecting statutory regulation for HCAs, the New Labour Government working party on workforce occupational regulation stated in 2009 that such a model 'was likely to be disproportionate to the risks involved and risked constraining roles and functions' (Department of Health, 2009a: 35). Similarly the Conservative-Led Coalition (CLC) has noted that 'In many cases, the risks to service users and the general public posed by groups of unregulated health and social care workers is not considered to be such that regulation of individual workers is necessary' (Department of Health, 2011: 16).

NHS Trusts perhaps most keen to ensure the cost efficient and flexible use of HCAs, have voiced their support for such a government approach. As the NHS Employers organization stressed in relation to the New Labour working party report (NHS Employers, 2009):

> We believe NHS organisations will agree with the underlying assumption about regulation in the report (inter alia) that if some form of regulation is required the solution should be the lightest possible touch.

The tensions between low-cost and high service quality in the use of HCAs have entered a particularly intense phase as new financial pressures on the NHS begin to take their effect. Between 2000–2010, government spending on the NHS increased by 70 per cent from £60 billion to £102 billion, with around 40 per cent spent on services provided by acute and foundation hospitals. Such an increase in expenditure was accompanied by an increased scrutiny over the returns received for such investment, with a growing concern about declining levels of productivity. Figures produced by the Office for National Statistics suggest that over this ten-year period productivity fell across the NHS by an average of 0.2% a year, and by an average of 1.4 per cent a year in hospitals. These concerns prompted the development of a Quality Innovation, Productivity and Protection programme in 2010 committed to delivering up to £20 billion of efficiency savings by 2014–2015. The pressures invoked by such a programme have been deepened by a sharp slowdown in public expenditure. Over this same four years, NHS funding will rise by £10 billion, the equivalent of a 0.1% a year increase in real terms. However, this is likely to be experienced as a real fall in funding: inflation is generally acknowledged as higher in the NHS than in the general economy, and demands on the NHS will increase over this period.

In such circumstances workforce structures and ways of working are likely to face increasing pressure. This reflects the fact that staffing costs represent around 40 per cent of total NHS costs: in 2007/2008 the total cost of all NHS staff in England was £36.5 billion and the total budget for the NHS that year was £90.4 billion (King's Fund, 2010). The link between this expenditure squeeze, staffing cuts, and care quality has already been highlighted by the RCN in its 'Frontline First' campaign. It has calculated that between April 2010 and November 2011 over 48,000 posts were set to be cut, half of this figure constituting clinical jobs. As RCN General Secretary Peter Carter has noted (RCN, 2011a): 'Cutting staff numbers … will undoubtedly have a deep and potentially dangerous impact on patient care'.

The interplay between the use of HCAs as a means of addressing cost and quality issues becomes even more apparent in a detailed consideration of the public policy objectives underpinning their use. The HCA role has been seen as a vehicle for the pursuit of various public policy objectives throughout much of the period of public expenditure growth under New Labour government as well as during the period of financial constraints under the CLC. Across this period of 15 years and with varying degrees of explicitness, four main public policy goals can be distinguished (Kessler et al., 2005), reflecting the HCA use as:

- a relief;
- a substitute;
- an apprentice; and
- a co-producer.

This chapter assesses these underlying objectives in two main sections. The first describes the policy goals in greater detail, exploring their source and rationale. The second unpacks the objectives, considering whether they are well founded and viable given the extant research literature.

Relief

As a relief HCAs have been seen by policymakers as a means of reducing the time spent by nurses on 'routine' or 'burdensome' tasks, so allowing them to concentrate on new or core professional activities. The use of the HCA in these terms might be seen as part of a broader move to restructure workforces in different parts of the public services, with a view to 'freeing-up' the professional. This was most clearly illustrated in primary and secondary education, where the Workload Agreement, 2004, re-allocated certain administrative tasks to the teaching assistant. The government explicitly repeated this approach in the children and families social care workforce, noting its intention 'to support employers and local service planners to remodel the workforce to enable social workers to concentrate on the complex work that needs their skills'.

In acute healthcare, the attempts to use the HCA in this way have been reflected in more fragmented and organic attempts to relieve the nurse of 'burdens' and 'routines'. The structure of the nursing and wider healthcare workforce is far more complex than in education and social care, lending itself less easily to restructuring. Governments have, however, taken a number of initiatives which might be seen to foster the HCA as a nurse relief. For example, they have developed a number of new roles or revived some older ones with this aim specifically in mind. The most striking is the housekeeper role, announced as part of the NHS Plan in 2000. As the initial guidance on this role, published by NHS Estates (2001) noted, it was 'being introduced across the NHS to release nurses from non-clinical tasks, such as chasing maintenance requests and to allow them to concentrate on nursing duties'. With a dedicated focus on cleaning, catering, and maintaining the environment, take-up of this housekeeper role by Trusts was uneven (May and Smith, 2003), but around a third of Trusts did have one by 2003, with nearly 5000 in post.

A more strategic response, the closest to the re-structuring initiatives in education and social care, took the form of the Modernising Nursing Careers (MNC) programme. Launched in 2006, this programme had a number of implications for the HCA role, and certainly sought to sharpen roles and lines of responsibility. The centrepiece of MNC was five proposed (career) pathways: children, family, and public health; first contact, access, and urgent care; supporting long-term care; acute and critical care; and mental health and psychosocial care. Cutting across these discrete pathways was the NHS career framework, establishing standard career levels (Department of Health, 2007b: 11). At levels 1–4 was the 'Associate', the new title for the assistant role, and responsible for 'supporting health, self care and care delivery'. At levels 5–7 was the Registered Nurse, 'leading care delivery, care co-ordination and case management'. At levels 8 and 9 was the Senior Registered Nurse, engaged in 'advance practice-delivery total care packages and complete episodes'.

However, the attempt to establish clinical career pathways and clarify stand-ard career levels and roles within each lacked explicit detail on the relationship between associates and registered nurses, with perhaps a mixed message being sent on the extent to which the former would relieve the latter of more routine tasks. The presentation of the nurse as a 'leader' and 'co-ordinator' within the MNC framework, suggested an enhanced delegation of tasks to the associate or assistant. Indeed, MNC (Department of Health 2006b: 15) highlighted the 'increased number of assistant roles as part of the multidisciplinary team' in describing the new nursing model. At the same time, however, there were some signs of a 'backlash' against such delegation and the deepening of nurse technical and specialist capabilities. Thus MNC also appeared to be seeking a 'better balance' between '(registered nurse) generalists and specialists'. In this respect it was seeking to encourage some nurses to re-engage with basic care activities.

Notwithstanding these tensions in MNC, a consistent strain within public policy has presented the HCA as available to take over from nurses some of the regular and standard chores related to direct and basic patient care, sometimes referred to as 'activities of daily living', such as washing, bed making, and feed-ing. As the Department of Health (2003a) noted, citing an example:

> Extending the role of the HCA has saved many hours of qualified nursing time. For example developing the competencies of HCAs on the stroke unit at Bradford (NHS Trust) has saved many hours of qualified nurse time.

Substitute

If policymakers have come to view the HCA as a relief taking over more rou-tine responsibilities from the nurse, the notion of the HCA as a substitute sees the role as encroaching more directly on traditional core nurse tasks. Once again there have been echoes of the assistant-as-substitute in other parts of the public services. In education, for example, the creation of the higher level teaching assistant (HLTA) with 'whole class responsibilities', such as covering for teacher absence, under the Workload Agreement was seen by some as a major incursion into the territory of the qualified teacher. Indeed, the develop-ment of the HLTA resulted in the National Union of Teachers refusing to sign this agreement. In nursing, the issue of professional territory has been equally, if not more, to the fore, and arguably the subject of longer-standing debate.

Much of this debate has revolved around the nature of nursing as a profes-sion, and where the core of the role actually lies. For some the nurse profession is advanced by the acquisition and deepening of technical and complex tasks and responsibilities. Many professions have been developed in this way, and in such a context the delegation of routine tasks become essential to an ever sharper focus on more specialized and difficult tasks. However, there has been an equally strong strain within nursing which suggests that any claim to professional status rests on the holistic provision of care: the notion that the nurse should deal with the patient 'in the round', addressing all of their needs from the most basic to the most complex. The UKCC Project 2000 report implied such an approach: as we saw, HCAs were only reluctantly presented as a nurse support given the practical barriers to the ideal of an all-registered nurse workforce. From such a holistic perspective the delegation of even the most routine tasks becomes problematic.

Some of these concerns about nurses taking on more specialist tasks and roles and leaving behind the holistic provision of care have recently been voiced by leaders within the profession. As the NHS Chief Nursing Officer (Department of Health, 2003b) warned:

> I believe that we are guilty of seeing caring as lower status as reflected in our keenness to delegate caring aspects of our role to others. Our actions fail to legitimise the value of caring – as nursing develops we tend to take on the roles and tasks from the medical profession.

Indeed, following a vote at the Royal College of Nursing Conference in 2004 *against* devolving the caring component of nursing to the HCA, the organization's General Secretary stated (BBC, 2004):

> If I become too posh to wash, I should no longer be in the profession. We are doing more than that. We are assessing the patient, we are doing holistic care, we are checking their emotional state.

These debates within nursing about the nature of the profession should not, however, detract from public policy developments which have sought to promote the HCA as a substitute for the nurse. These developments have taken different forms. In part they can be seen in the promotion of new nurse support roles, most obviously the assistant practitioner at Band 4. Thus, Skills for Health (2011) in its definition of the AP, very clearly sees it as taking on core nurse tasks:

> The Assistant Practitioners would be able to deliver elements of health and social care and undertake clinical work in domains that have *previously only been within the remit of registered professionals*. The assistant practitioner may transcend professional boundaries. [Emphasis added.]

More broadly, there has been a renewed interest in skill mix, in particular whether and to what degree unregistered HCAs might safely be traded-off against registered nurses in the composition of the nursing workforce. It is an issue which has been linked with shortages in the supply of registered nurses over the years, but more particularly the use of HCAs has been noted in the context of budgetary constraints: they have been seen as a 'cheaper' option to nurses (Grimshaw, 1999). In contrast to a number of developed countries where there are mandatory skill mix ratios, hospitals in Britain have had considerable discretion on this aspect of staffing. This has given rise to a considerable prescriptive research literature on approaches to establishing 'a safe' skill mix (Scott, 2003). As already implied, this has been seen as heavily contingent upon a range of factors, although the RCN in 2006 set a benchmark 'headline' registered/unregistered ratio of 65/35 (RCN, 2006).

Given the contemporary financial challenges facing the NHS it is unsurprising that skill mix has re-emerged as a key issue for policymakers and practitioners (Nursing Times, 2007). As Gerry O'Dwyer, senior employment adviser at the RCN, has noted (Nursing Times, 2009a): 'If we are dealing with £15 to £20 billion (in reduced cost) you don't save that by not providing biscuits at board meetings. It's length of stay, productivity and skill mix'. In such circumstances the pressure might well be towards more diluted forms of skill mix, a possibility implicitly flagged-up in a report by the consultancy firm McKinsey in 2007 when it questioned any moves towards mandatory ratios (The Guardian, 2010). Indeed, the *Nursing Times* (2009b) reports that 'a number of NHS hospitals are planning to replace an increasing number of trained nurses with cheaper unregistered staff'.

Apprentice

As an 'apprentice', the HCA role has been seen by policymakers as a means of strengthening workforce capacity. This might be achieved in two ways. The first relies on individuals developing within the HCA role, in effect becoming more capable HCAs, and as a consequence moving up the unregistered career and pay band levels. The second views HCAs as representing a future potential supply of registered nurses, not least in the light of periodic shortages, using the role as a stepping stone into the profession. The HCA role has value in these respects in that it is perceived as being a particularly stable element of the workforce. Indeed the use of the HCA role as an apprentice is often associated with a 'grow-your-own' approach to the workforce. As Malhotra notes in a King's Fund report (2006: 2) 'grow-your-own workforce strategies are characterised by ... looking to local labour markets as a key source of workforce supply [and] by encouraging organisations to use the skills and talent of their existing unregistered workforce more effectively'.

The development of the HCA-as-apprentice can be related to a broader stream of public policy over the last decade or so, progressively deepened in the NHS. From the outset the New Labour government (1997–2010) attached considerable importance to lifelong learning. This included an emphasis on access to the professions, reflected in a government-commissioned report by Alan Langlands in 2005 on this issue. In important respects the NHS was ahead of this agenda, placing considerable weight on learning and development opportunities for HCAs. We have seen that the restructuring of the nursing workforce following Project 2000 was accompanied by moves to accredit HCA capabilities on the basis of NVQ qualifications. Moreover, there have been long-standing secondment schemes, providing opportunities for HCAs to be supported in training as registered nurses. These fragmented initiatives were placed on a firmer, more structured basis in an NHS Framework for Lifelong Learning. As the government noted (Department of Health, 2001: 17):

> We want to open up opportunities for people who join NHS organisations at relatively low skill levels to progress their skills through investment in their training and development to professional levels and beyond.

The infrastructure for the career and personal development of those performing the HCA role (and indeed other NHS roles) coalesced around the notion of the 'Skills Escalator' (Department of Health, 2007c). Comprising a collection of systems, the Skills Escalator was based upon a number of principles and elements. It sought to achieve transparency and achievable career pathways. Work roles had to be based upon clearly articulated competencies. These competencies needed to be accredited and delivered by an educational provider, with an educational pathway established by which the individual could acquire them, so establishing their capability to perform the work role.

Attention has already been drawn to a number of developments across the NHS and designed to take forward this agenda, in particular the NHS Career Framework and Agenda for Change underpinned by the Knowledge and Skills framework. These general developments, in turn, were more explicitly harnessed to attempts to develop those in HCA roles. Indeed, the importance of this focus on the HCA-as-apprentice in taking forward other public policy goals, such as the HCA-as-relief, is made explicit in the government's (Department of Health, 2003a) observation that:

> As existing staff develop into new roles on the skills escalator, so the time of more highly skilled staff can be used more effectively. For instance suitably skilled support workers could carry out some of the current tasks of registered nurses, freeing up these nurses to contribute more fully with their skills. The new pay system will recognise those roles and provide incentives for staff to acquire necessary extra skills.

More specifically interest in the development of this apprentice dimension was apparent in the Thames Gateway Project, (Skills for Health, 2009) funded by the government as part of its response to the Langlands report and specifically seeking to facilitate the learning and development of those on Agenda for Change pay bands 1–4. Commencing in 2007 and reporting in 2009 this project was taken forward by the Department of Health's Widening Participation in Learning Strategy Unit, under the label of 'Growing our own professions in the new NHS.' It was work which culminated in a Skills for Health framework, providing guidance to both NHS organizations and employees on how those in pay bands 1–4 might be developed. This extended from helping organizations build a business case for such developments to highlighting how the individual learner might be supported.

Co-producer

The final public policy objective informing the development of the HCA role views it as contributing in a distinctive way to the provision of healthcare: HCAs are co-producing by bringing to the ward team particular and unique qualities. In contrast to the HCA as a relief or a substitute, models which imply a significant overlap between HCA and nurse roles, as a co-producer the HCA is seen as providing added value to the quality of care in its own right. As the then Health Minister John Denham (Hansard, 1999) noted:

> HCAs are an invaluable and important part of the NHS … they make an important contribution to the direct care of patients *as well as* supporting a range of professionals in a wide variety of ways. [Emphasis added.]

It is striking here that reference is being made to an HCA contribution to direct care 'as well as' providing professional support. It suggests that HCAs have a distinctive contribution to make over and above such support. It was a view more recently and explicitly stated in the Next Stage Review (Department of Health, 2008):

> A key priority for the Next Stage Review is the development of the workforce, including those in clinical support roles, to deliver high quality and safe care. The wider healthcare team is essential both to the modernisation of professional career frameworks and to the quality of patient experience. They have continual and regular contact with patients and provide essential support to multi-disciplinary teams in the delivery of care.

The distinctive HCA contribution might be seen to derive from two sources: the nature of the role and the types of individuals performing it. The HCA role sits beneath the registered role in the healthcare occupational hierarchy and as such might be perceived as more accessible and less intimidating to the patient. Structured in this way, it might also be regarded as attractive to individuals with a different personal profile to other members of the ward team, one perhaps filled by people who more easily relate to and reflect the background of the patient.

The 'added value' of the HCA role and its post holders has not always been easily or readily acknowledged by the nursing profession. In this form the role has perhaps been seen as a challenge to the nurses' status. Indeed, more generally, the nurse profession has sometimes found it difficult to position itself in relation to the HCA. As already suggested, the nurse support role presents a threat to professional boundaries, encouraging some in the profession to emphasize and accentuate status and role differences. The language used in the past to discuss HCAs is interesting in this respect. Writing about the development of the nurse auxiliary role in the late 1970s, Johnson, without a touch of irony, sounds a note of warning to the nursing profession, 'Authority must command respect, and there are some grounds for believing that the workers on the ground floor of nursing are breaking out of their traditional deference'.

More significantly, these concerns have been reflected in how the RCN has engaged with HCAs. The general public services union, UNISON, has remained the main recruiter of HCAs, with the RCN moving only gradually to admitting this group as members. It was only in October 2011 that HCAs, as 'health practitioners', were allowed full membership of the RCN, following the failure of a similar motion the year before. Previously, HCAs were only allowed to become associate members of the college with no representation on the RCN council. Under the new arrangements they have a similar status to student nurses, voting for two council representatives.

In summary, it has been suggested that national public policymakers have come to view the HCA role in a number of guises, designed to pursue different objectives: as a relief, relieving registered nurses of 'burdensome' routines and allowing them to concentrate on core activities; as a substitute, taking on more of the core activities, perhaps in a more cost efficient way; as an apprentice, adding to workforce capacity by developing within the role, or moving into registered nursing; and as a co-producer, making a distinctive contribution to patient care.

The achievement of these objectives is, however, founded upon a series of assumptions. As Figure 2.1 indicates, these assumptions fall within four research domains and take a number of forms:

• HCAs as a strategic resource;
• The personal backgrounds and characteristics of HCAs;
• The shape and nature of the HCA role;
• The consequences of the HCA role.

The next section considers these assumptions and the evidence for them. It argues that, at best, this evidence base is fragmented and patchy.

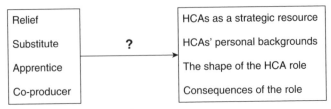

Figure 2.1 Objectives and assumptions.

Policy assumptions and the current evidence base

Over the years, a significant body of research on the nurse support role in Britain and in other developed countries has emerged covering the four domains of interest distinguished in Figure 2.1. Table A1 in the Appendix provides a schematic overview of the academic research specifically undertaken on HCAs (other broader studies have sometimes touched in passing on HCAs, but these are not included in Table A1) highlighting the research focus and questions, the methods adopted, and the main findings. This overview reveals a number of features of the academic research 'canon' on HCAs:

- Much of the research has been conducted by researchers in university nursing or health studies departments, and published in nursing journals. There appears to have been much more limited research work on HCAs in other disciplines, say organization studies, employment relations, and the sociology of work.

- In terms of substantive focus, there has been a marked focus on how different stakeholders view the HCA role: ward managers, registered nurses, and HCAs themselves. There has been some shared interest in a number of other topics: HCAs' experience of moving into nursing; the work undertaken by HCAs; and how HCA work relates to that of nurses. Intensive care settings emerge as quite a popular setting for assessing the HCA role.

- Methodologically, many of the studies are small scale, both in terms of participants and organizations covered. There is an emphasis on qualitative research approaches, interviews in the main, unsurprising given the strong interest in perceptions of the HCA role. This should not detract from a few more intense multi-method cases, and surveys covering a wide spread of organizations or units.

- Research has generated descriptions of many aspects of the HCA role, but given its limited connection to any broader analytical frameworks and debates, there is little explanation as to how and why the role has developed and with what impact.

This section draws upon the academic research outlined in the Appendix, and other material, to explore the extant evidence for assumptions informing the public policy goals underpinning the use of HCAs. In so doing, it also seeks to develop a sharper set of research issues and questions which might be taken forward for analysis. Primarily the focus remains on British findings: as already noted in Chapter 1, the idiosyncratic and path-dependent nature of the nurse support role in this country suggests the need for some care in assuming the applicability or relevance of research work from other national contexts. The four research domains from Figure 2.1 are considered in turn.

The HCA as a strategic resource

The presentation of the HCA role as a means of addressing a range of public policy objectives assumes the propensity of NHS Trusts and other relevant institutions to act strategically in terms of workplace planning across the nursing workforce, and specifically in relation to the development and use of the HCA role. If the HCA is to be used to help modify the nurse role, to address future staffing needs, or to improve the quality of the patient experience, it suggests the need for an explicit, coherent, and planned Trust-wide approach to the role. Whether or not the HCA role is being considered by Trusts in these strategic terms remains unclear; this is in part a consequence of opaque systems for planning the nursing workforce, but also the result of limited research exploring this issue.

In the main, systems for planning the nursing workforce have functioned at the regional level, typically linked to the commissioning of nurse training places, but subject to regular change over the years, not least a consequence of frequent organizational modifications to this tier of the NHS. Most recently, such planning was principally undertaken by the Strategic Health Authority (SHA), 'with lead responsibility to support the assessment of workforce requirements within their geographic areas, in association with NHS employers at trust level' (Buchan, 2007). General workforce planning in the NHS has, however, been subject to considerable recent criticism, particularly by the House of Commons Health Committee (House of Commons Health Committee, 2007), which pointed to the need for a system better able to integrate medical and non-medical workforce planning and to deliver a more flexible workforce. This view is supported by the research of Imison et al. (2009), who, in reviewing the existing workforce strategies and investment plans of SHAs, found that seven out of ten were investing less than 5 per cent of their budget on training linked to new ways of working and new roles.

This set-up suggests that individual Trusts have had limited in-house resource and capacity to explore the use and development of the HCA role.

There have, however, been few, if any, attempts to examine the strategic use of the HCA in the research literature. The closest the research community has come to dealing with this issue is work on skill mix at Trust level. This literature suggests that rather than adopting a strategic approach, Trusts have been opportunistic in their engagement with the HCA role, reflected in a shifting balance between registered and non-registered staff as a response to changing financial circumstances (Roberts, 1995). This expediency has been seen to extend to the manipulation of grade mix (Grimshaw, 1999), with some Trusts seeking to use locally graded and cheaper HCAs as a replacement for the national nurse auxiliary grade to save costs.

Within the context of current workforce planning constraints, and given the absence of recent research, it remains worth considering whether and how senior Trust managers have engaged with the HCA role as part of a more strategic approach to the workforce. Has the current system squeezed out opportunities for Trusts to consider the role in these terms or is there residual scope to do so?

Backgrounds

If HCAs are seen as a potential source for future registered nurses, as a relief or substitute for nurses, and as providing a distinctive contribution to patient care, the background characteristics of those taking up the job become crucial: do those entering the role have the requisite skills, aspirations, and motivation to give effect to these policy goals? Do post holders want to become nurses or to develop within the role? Do they bring to the HCA role capabilities from previous paid or unpaid work roles and a disposition which impacts on how they perform within it?

Over the years, an increasingly detailed picture has emerged of the personal characteristics of HCAs, particularly drawing on the regular surveys conducted by Thornley (1997) and UNISON (2008). Such surveys and others (Knibb et al., 2006) have highlighted the gendered nature of the role, most post holders being relatively mature women, sometimes working part-time and with ongoing domestic responsibilities. Some insight has also been provided into the aspirations of HCAs, the UNISON survey (2008) suggested considerable interest amongst these employees in undertaking nursing or other professional training.

Data on the background of HCAs, however, remain limited in a number of respects. First, there is a paucity of qualitative data which might provide a greater in-depth appreciation of the factors that lead individuals to the HCA role: what are entrants seeking from it and how do their lives beyond the 'hospital gates' shape what they do within them? Second, there is little hard data on the past working patterns of HCAs; what kinds of sectors and occupations are they drawn from, and which employment experiences provide gateways into the role? Third, there is a marked absence of material on how local labour markets and the general demographics of an area affect the supply and kinds of people taking up the HCA role. Attention has been drawn to considerable regional variation in vacancy rates in a range of healthcare occupations within the NHS (Healthcare Commission, 2005). As Elliott et al. (2003) note 'the nature of characteristics of the local labour market [are] crucial in shaping Trusts' responses to [staff] shortage and in turn their competitiveness'. Fourth, there have been very few attempts to contrast HCA backgrounds with those of nurses: an important means of defining the HCA lies in distinguishing them from the nurse in background terms.

The shape and nature of the HCA role

In presenting the HCA as both a potential relief and a substitute for the nurse, policymakers are making profound assumptions, not only about the general form assumed by the role, but more specifically about its capacity to embrace tasks which range from the routine to the more technically sophisticated. The notion of an extended HCA role has long been acknowledged amongst practitioners. As Hardie (1978) observed over 30 years ago in relation to the nursing auxiliary, 'work can vary from some basic nursing skills, such as bed making and maintenance of equipment, to dealing with complex interpersonal and technical situations'. However, within the context of recent policy pronouncements, questions are raised about the shape of the contemporary HCA role. These questions relate to the nature of the tasks performed and how these are packaged, as well as to the form assumed by any extension of the role.

Much previous research on the nurse support role has focused on the tasks and activities undertaken, considering them in a number of different ways. First, the HCA role has been explored in different healthcare settings, with a particular interest in general practice (Bosley and Dale, 2008), intensive care units both within acute (Hogan and Playle, 2000) and community mental healthcare (Meek, 1998), as well as in general hospital wards (Spilsbury, 2004; Spilsbury and Meyer, 2004; Knibb et al., 2006). While these studies have adopted different methodologies, from the nationwide survey (Hogan and Playle, 2000) to the in-depth case study (Spilsbury and Meyer, 2004), one of the more common findings relates to the ongoing fluidity, variation, and, in some instances, uncertainty in the use of the role. The various forms assumed by the role might well have implications for its capacity to pursue different public policy goals. For example, Wakefield et al. (2009) find that depending on the nature of the assistant practitioner role, it might be used both as a means of assistance to the nurse, in our terms relieving them of certain tasks, or as a means of substitution, undertaking the tasks of the registered nurse.

Second, researchers have explored the shape of the role by reference to the frequency with which different tasks are undertaken by the HCA, often with a view to identifying the degree of overlap with the registered nurse role. Survey work (Thornley, 1997; Knibb et al., 2006) has highlighted the propensity for most HCAs to undertake certain basic tasks such as bed making and patient bathing while also noting the performance of more complex and technical tasks associated with, for example, dressings and catheters. Indeed, Thornley (2000) stresses a marked similarity in the activities undertaken by HCAs and nurses, implying that, in practice, differences in the contours of the respective roles should not be overstated.

Third, there have been attempts to examine the shape of the role as viewed by various stakeholders. This work has tended to drift into the prescriptive; for example, ward managers at one large Acute Trust had highlighted the need to further extend the HCA role (Jack et al., 2004), while radiology service managers in the south of England stressed the importance of HCAs given shortages in radiographers (Ford, 2004).

Previous research, then, has provided important insights into the general shape of the HCA role in a number of different healthcare settings, while at the same time suggesting that it is not an easy role to 'tie down'; the role appears to take various forms, extending across a range of tasks in different combinations, sometimes overlapping with work of the registered nurses. It is a view of the role which opens up two key issues: one linked to the forms assumed by the role, and the other to the factors shaping them.

There is a need for a sharper conceptualization and characterization of the HCA role which captures its different manifestations. What patterns can be distinguished in the shape of the HCA role? In the context of the general debate on the possible extension of the HCA role, where does the core of the role lie, and, given the longevity of the nurse support role, has this core shifted? Addressing such questions requires an in-depth evaluation of the tasks performed by HCAs, designed to pick up variation in a nuanced way. For example, while past research has often asked whether or not given tasks are undertaken, a more variegated picture might emerge if consideration was given to *how often* they were performed: a role which involves the occasional performance of a task is a very different to one where a task is routinely undertaken.

If the HCA role takes different forms, it follows that analysis of how and why these forms have emerged is also required. A distinction between structure and agency is useful in this respect. This distinction has been core to debates in social theory, with views varying on the explanatory value of the two.

Structure relates to institutions, in the form of a stable set of rules or practices, which determine in a fairly mechanistic way individual and collective attitudes and behaviours. Agency is predicated on the autonomy of the individual or the collective to make choices and exercise a high degree of discretion. The exercise of structure and agency has been theorized in different ways. These have often been presented as mutually exclusive, with one being privileged over the other. But this is not necessarily the case: some have suggested that agency might be constrained but not determined by structure.

In the current context, the structure–agency distinction raises questions about the balance between the two in shaping the HCA role. In exploring the role in different healthcare settings, the importance of structural context is implied but rarely explored; there have been few attempts to compare the role between settings or between organizations in the same setting, or even between, say, different clinical areas in the same organization. The limited attention paid to structure in these terms is surprising given a possible link between institutional context and the HCA role. Healthcare setting and clinical area might well be expected to influence the type of patient cared for and the tasks therefore performed. The different work systems, cultures, and management styles of the Trust or of lower level organizational units such as the division or ward, might similarly be assumed to have an impact upon the nature of the role.

The potency of individual agency against this backdrop remains an interesting empirical question (Spilsbury, 2004). The research interest in the individual backgrounds and aspirations of HCAs suggests that agency has residual significance, and yet few researchers have investigated the link between agency, the shape of the HCA role, and performance within it.

Consequences
For the HCA

The public policy objectives underpinning the use of HCAs have very different and potentially contradictory consequences for those individuals actually performing the role. As a relief, the HCA is presented as acquiring the more mundane tasks which, while freeing up the nurse, conjures up the spectre of a degraded job. Moreover, in viewing the HCA as a substitute, questions are raised about the 'fairness' of a situation where HCAs are undertaking traditional nurse tasks on a considerably lower wage. On the other hand, as an apprentice, the HCA is seen as having opportunities for career development either within or beyond the role, holding out the hope of improvements in the present and future quality of working life.

Research on the degradation or enrichment of the HCA's working life has placed greater emphasis on the former. Views on the nature of the degradation have, however, varied. First, a stream of research has emphasized an undervaluing of the HCA role over the years, seen as deriving from certain biases in formal pay and grading systems. Thornley (1996, 2002) has noted the lack of sensitivity in such systems to the kind of tacit, caring skills which HCAs typically bring to the role, leading to a consistent under-rewarding. Second, work has highlighted certain grievances held by HCAs about working relationships. In part, this is reflected in a perceived misuse of the HCA by nurses (Spilsbury and Meyer, 2004) but has also been seen to derive from some uncertainty amongst nurses as to how to use HCAs efficiently and effectively (Workman, 1996). Third, research has suggested a more general disillusionment with the role, reflected in a survey of UNISON's HCA members (UNISON, 2008), which showed that around a third of respondents had 'seriously considered leaving the role', many because they 'felt under-valued by the employer'. Fourth, researchers have cast some doubt on the willingness and ability of HCAs to take advantage of the career development opportunities associated with the role, a function of the practical difficulties individuals face in undertaking further training (Gould et al., 2006). Research highlighting negative outcomes for post holders has tended to eclipse work noting more positive consequences. However, Knibb et al. (2006), using an established job satisfaction scale, report fairly positive HCA views on working conditions, while Cox et al. (2008), in a study on the Skills Escalator find some extension of career opportunities for NHS support workers, albeit unevenly distributed across the country.

The suggestion that the HCA role has mixed consequences for post holders encourages a further consideration of outcomes. This might involve a more thorough consideration of the factors which influence HCAs' work experience, while also elaborating on the ways in which impact is assessed. One measure generally overlooked by researchers relates to the emotional impact of the HCA role on those who perform it. Caring work as a form of emotional labour has attracted considerable research interest in recent years (Hochschild, 1983) and yet while nursing has consistently been seen as an example of such labour (Theodosius, 2008), HCAs have rarely been considered in these terms. There are strong grounds for arguing that the emotional consequences of care work in an acute setting are likely to be as, if not more, intense for the HCA than for the nurse: with HCAs increasingly taking on the direct care work, the emotional fallout from such care is likely to fall disproportionately on those within the role.

For the nurse

The public policy objectives which view the HCA as a relief, a substitute, and a co-producer also have contradictory implications for the nurse. These connect

to some of the ambiguities underpinning the pursuit of nurse professionalization. As a relief, the HCA would appear to be of straightforward benefit to the
nurse. The literature on professionalization has long highlighted the value of a
lower-order occupational group to the would-be profession. Abbott (1988)
views such support roles as available to professionals to take on 'dangerously
routine work' which otherwise might dilute claims to knowledge-based expertise. As Hughes (1993) has noted in a healthcare context, 'Nurses, as they successfully rise to professional standing, are delegating the more lowly of their
traditional tasks to aides and maids'.

On closer inspection, however, a number of potential difficulties for the
nurse flow from the HCA role. The first lies in the other policy objectives highlighted for the role. As a substitute and a co-producer, HCAs might be seen to
represent a threat to nurses and their jurisdictions; in the case of the former by
taking over their core tasks and, in relation to the latter by bringing distinctive
capabilities to bear on patient care. Allen (2001: 81) has highlighted the 'boundary work' undertaken by the registered nurse to protect their jurisdictions, for
example, the recounting of 'cautionary tales' on the extended use of HCAs. In
a policy context, these concerns have been reflected in a traditional reluctance
on the part of the RCN to admit nurse support workers into membership. As
Rye (1978) noted some years ago, 'There is no doubt that if the RCN is to
retain its credibility as a professional organization, it cannot receive into membership untrained personnel who are not training for any of the statutory
qualifications'. As noted earlier, it is an approach which the RCN have only
relatively recently changed.

The second difficulty for nurses as a discreet occupational group resides in
competing notions of nursing as a profession (Doherty, 2007). As noted, the
HCA as a relief supports a model of nurse professionalization based upon the
delegation of routine tasks as more technical and specialist tasks are acquired.
However, for those who view claims to professional status as resting on the
provision of holistic nursing care, the casting-off of the apparently routine
becomes more problematic.

This concern is reflected in the ambiguity of the RCN to nurse engagement
with direct, basic caring tasks as part of holistic care: as nurses readily take
on advanced nurse roles with implications for their ability to perform
such tasks, the RCN is voting against devolving the caring component of
nursing to HCAs. As the then General Secretary stated in the wake of this
2004 vote:

> We [nurses] are assessing the patient, we are doing holistic care, we are checking their
> emotional state ... I don't know how you can talk about caring and nursing. It's the
> same thing. Nursing to me is caring.

The third potential difficulty for nurses with the HCA role lies in the realm of management and accountability. The HCA remains a member of the ward team who has to be managed within the context of ongoing nurse responsibility for patient care. The NMC code of practice is clear on this issue, noting that nurses are responsible for the delegation of tasks but not for the performance of the tasks themselves. However, in the mind of the busy nurse, this distinction might not always be easily drawn. Uncertainty and caution on their part would be understandable: HCAs are not regulated so denying nurses any default quality assurance on HCAs' capabilities and it is, after all, nurse registration that is 'on the line' for any error of judgement.

This uncertainty about nurse accountability has been heightened by the high-profile cases of healthcare failure associated with skill mix issues, and might well explain the increasingly shrill calls from the nurse establishment to regulate the HCA role. Certainly, it is a concern which has prompted the RCN to devote considerable resources to publicizing and clarifying how registered nurses stand in these terms: in 2011 it produced a guidance booklet and video, *Accountability and delegations: What you need to know* (RCN, 2011b), which set out the principles of accountability and delegation for nurses, students, HCAs, and assistant practitioners.

Research on nurse engagement with HCAs has touched upon some of these issues. There is some evidence to suggest that HCAs have effectively relieved nurses of certain routine activities allowing them to focus on core professional tasks (Power et al., 1990). Unsurprisingly perhaps, this has encouraged a positive nurse view of the HCA role (Reeve, 1994). At the same time, there are data to suggest some tension in this relationship. McKenna (2004) revealed that nurses were devoting a growing amount of time to inducting, training, and supervising increasing numbers of HCAs, a finding echoed in a survey of UK nurses. McLaughlin et al. (2000) found 'some concern regarding RN delegation and supervision to nursing care assistants that occasionally distracted from RN duties'.

A number of studies have also highlighted continued nurse attempts to protect their occupational jurisdiction and to resist HCA encroachment in the form of substitution. This is reflected in ongoing 'boundary work' performed by nurses, for example, in the form of atrocity stories (Dingwell, 1977; Bach et al., 2008) about HCAs' 'mistakes'; or in the way in which nursing roles are presented in HCA and nurse training and induction to retain a clear nurse–HCA demarcation (Allen, 2001).

These findings suggest a degree of ambivalence towards the HCA role on the part of registered nurses and their representative organizations, an orientation which might well reflect some of the tensions highlighted in nurse profession-alization strategies (Daykin and Clarke, 2000). It is an ambivalence which encourages further evaluation of the HCA from the nurse perspective: wheth-er, when, and why the role is viewed in a positive or negative light.

For the patient

For the patient, the double-edged impact of the HCA role lies in very different possibilities as to its effect on the quality of care. As a relief taking on much of the direct patient care from nurses and as a substitute taking on more technical tasks, issues related to HCA capability and the possible dilution of service standards emerge, often coalescing around concerns about risk and safety. Yet as a co-producer, the HCA role, at a lower level to the nurse and perhaps filled by those with very different sorts of backgrounds to the professional, has the potential to provide a less intimidating and more empathic form of care. These assumed consequences for the patient of the HCA role have a weak evidence base, and once again the limited research undertaken has generated far from conclusive findings.

McKenna et al. (2004) are forthright in their concern about the use of HCAs from a patient perspective, asserting that 'the increasing reliance on HCAs raises serious quality and safety questions'. Such worries find an echo in a sur-vey of chief executives in health and social care organizations which found that over half (52%) felt that there was a 'considerable' or 'moderate' risk from the use of such employees (Saks et al., 2007). The most significant stream of rele-vant research has focused on the relationship between skill mix and clinical patient outcomes, raising questions about the impact on the quality of care as more HCAs are used relative to nurses. This research has consistently shown a positive relationship between the richness of the skill mix and such outcomes (Carr-Hill et al., 1992; McKenna, 1995), although there has been some criti-cism of such research, for example, its tendency to equate skill with grade and job title rather than exploring in greater detail the experience and capabilities nursing staff might bring to patient care (Spilsbury and Meyer, 2001).

These patient concerns have found recent expression, and been reinforced, by a storm of criticism about the quality of health and social care. Attention has already been drawn to the cases of Mid Staffordshire and Tunbridge Wells. More generally, there has been a series of additional developments, which in combination have created a sense of crisis in care delivery:

- Winterbourne View: in May 2011, the BBC *Panorama* programme revealed 'serious abuse and appalling standards of care' in a private hospital, Winterbourne View, for people with learning disabilities.

- A review of care for older people in 100 hospitals carried out by the Care Quality Commission in March and June 2011, indicated that well under half (45) were fully competent, with almost a quarter (20) non-compliant (CQC, 2011).
- A report by the Equality and Human Rights Commission into the provision of health and social care for older people in their homes, suggested that the quality of care was often so 'poor' that the dignity and rights of the elderly were being compromised (ERHC, 2011).
- At the end of 2011, the Department of Health, along with the National Audit Office and Common's Public Accounts Committee, commenced investigations into the Care Quality Commission, reviewing whether it was fit for purpose, not least given the instances highlighted above and its failure to pick them up.

This crisis in care has been related with varying degrees of explicitness to workforce issues, although with the provision of such care relying so much on the workforce it is hard to escape the conclusion that staffing issues have played a major part. The EHRC (2011: 73) is quite clear on this issue noting: 'Care workers are low paid, and may get little training and inadequate supervision and support ... There are no qualification requirements'. The 'problems' associated with the use of assistants are understated, but with much of this care provided by such workers doubts have been raised about their capabilities. Indeed, these doubts have been deepened by the more assertive and unambiguous worries highlighted by leaders from the nursing profession about support workers within the context of these broader care crisis.

Against this backdrop, it is, however, important to stress that research on whether HCAs add value to patient care is scarce. There have been suggestions that rather than undermining care quality, HCAs bring distinctive competencies to caring work. James (1992), for example, in her study of nursing in a hospice setting, stresses the skills nurse auxiliaries display in the context of emotional labour, which she defines in terms of managing the emotion of patients and their relatives: 'There is almost an inverse of status and skill in emotional labour ... young staff nurses relied on the four older auxiliaries who were described as being the backbone of the unit'. James relates this nurse reliance on auxiliaries in part to the auxiliaries' greater work experience, but also to the auxiliaries' tacit capabilities to manage the emotions of others, developed in a domestic environment and effectively brought to bear in an employment context.

The absence of research on the consequences of HCAs for patient care in an acute care setting in the light of policy assumptions is striking, particularly given the weight now placed on the role as the direct care provider. Basic but crucial questions have simply not been posed, let alone explored: whether patients can distinguish between HCAs and other members of the nursing team; whether patients develop a distinctive relationship with HCAs; and whether the nature of this relationship impacts on patient outcomes. Equally noteworthy has been the absence of the patient voice on this and other issues related to the HCA role.

Summary

It has been argued that policymakers have come to view the HCA role as an increasingly important vehicle for the pursuit of various public policy goals. The role has become crucial in the search for cost efficiency and service quality, being presented by policymakers as: a relief, reducing burdens on nurses; as a substitute, taking on core registered nurse tasks; as an apprentice increasing NHS workforce capacity by providing in-role development opportunities or routes into registered nursing; and as co-producer, the nature of the role and or its post holders making distinctive contributions to care delivery.

It has been stressed, however, that these aspirations are based on a number of often heroic assumptions about the role, those who perform it, and its impact. More specifically, these assumptions are related to four research domains: the use of HCAs as a strategic resource; the background of those individuals taking up the HCA post; the shape and nature of the HCA role; and the consequences of the role for various stakeholders. A review of the research literature on the HCA role suggested that the evidence base for these assumptions was at best patchy and uneven. Previous research had often been narrow, both in terms of substantive focus and methodological approach. Moreover, the exploration of these issues remained considerably under-theorized, with considerable scope to debate the plausibility of these policymaker assumptions. This was highlighted with reference to the possible impact of the role for different stakeholders, with various conceivable outcomes being presented. Thus the role was seen as possibly providing opportunities for the HCA, but equally condemning the post holder to a heavier, more routine workload. It was viewed as lending the registered nurse valued support, perhaps removing onerous burdens, whilst at the same time running the risk of adding to the nurses' management responsibility and diluting professional claims to the holistic provision of care. Finally, the role had the potential to provide patients with a more accessible, less intimidating source of care, and yet ran the risk of generating new concerns about safety and care quality.

The remainder of this book is devoted to a research study which sought to address the questions raised in our four research domains, in a structured and systematic way, and in so doing strengthen the evidence base for the use of the HCA role. In the next chapter we turn to this study, setting out a clear set of research questions and how we sought to address them.

Chapter 3

Research focus, design, and methods

Introduction

Building upon the foundations provided by the extant research literature, we sought to develop a study which:

- Addressed policy assumptions underpinning the use of HCAs. These assumptions related to the deployment of HCAs as a strategic resource. They also touched on HCA backgrounds and the tasks performed by post holders. Finally they were associated with the consequences of the role for various stakeholders.

- Not only described the HCA role and its outcomes, but also sought to theorize or provide plausible explanations for these developments.

- Provided a more in-depth understanding of who HCAs are and what they do, so heightening their visibility as an influence on the patient experience and, as a consequence, as an important contributor to Trust performance.

- Gave a voice to different actors with a stake in the role, particularly patients, an often overlooked stakeholder group.

- Present a comprehensive picture of the HCA role by drawing on various types of data and considering issues from different stakeholder perspectives.

This chapter is divided into four main sections aligned to these goals. The first section frames the research, clarifying its scope and the underpinning research questions along with an elaboration of how key terms have been conceptualized. The second sets out the analytical framework used to address these questions and the third details the research methods used and the nature of the data generated. The final section outlines the descriptive and analytical narratives shaping the presentation of the findings.

Framing the study: scope and research questions

The research was concerned with HCAs at Agenda for Change pay bands 2 and 3 in an acute or secondary healthcare setting. It did not, therefore, explore pay band 4 assistant practitioner roles. As we have seen, pay band 2 and 3 HCAs comprise the main body of the unregistered nurse support workforce, emerging from the nurse auxiliary role, previously graded A and B. While HCAs have increasingly been developed in community healthcare settings (Bosely and Dale, 2008), their presence is again more firmly established in an acute setting, and on a much more significant scale.

It is worth restating that the workers covered by the study conformed to the NMC HCA definition, therefore excluding ancillary workers such as porters and cleaners. Those workers providing administrative support, such as ward clerks, were also not covered in our research, falling outside of this definition. It was open to greater debate as to whether ward housekeepers were captured by the NMC definition; they were, however, again not covered in this research. Ward housekeepers were typically part of the ward team, and might have direct contact with patients, particularly at meal times. They were, however, directed mainly by the ward manager, rather than by the registered nurse. In some instances, ward housekeepers fell within the Trust's Estates rather than nursing directorate, in such cases generating managerial and supervisory tensions: the ward manager directing the housekeeper, whose first-line manager nonetheless lay outside of nursing in the estates and facilities department. In contrast to porters and cleaners, administrative staff and housekeepers are typically part of the ward teams, and whilst not dealt with directly in the research, they will be seen to have some bearing on the nature and use of HCA roles.

The research concentrated on the following questions:

To what extent have HCAs been viewed and used as a strategic resource by trusts in secondary healthcare?

This question sought to establish whether and how HCAs, as a discrete occupational group, had been considered and deployed by senior hospital managers in the pursuit of broad Trust objectives. This involved looking at whether the four public policy goals of relief, substitute, apprentice, and co-producer found any resonance in deliberations and practice at Trust level. This might have been reflected in, for example, considered attempts to recruit and retain HCAs, to train and develop them, or to use them in innovative and flexible ways with the explicit aim of improving the efficiency and effectiveness of patient care.

What are the backgrounds of those taking up the HCA role?

The background of those individuals taking up the HCA role was considered in demand and supply side terms. On the demand side, the kind of people attracted to the role was seen as affected by the formal requirements of the Trust, as reflected in entry criteria, person and job specifications, and less formally, in the actual practice of those Trust managers responsible for recruitment. On the supply side, various features assumed importance in characterizing HCA backgrounds:

- *Personal profile:* such features as age, ethnicity, domestic circumstances, and links to the local community, were seen as an influence on how individuals engaged with the HCA role, the latent and tacit skills they brought to it, and what they were seeking from it in the context of broader life needs and interests. A comparison with nurses was seen as particularly enlightening in establishing whether or not HCAs were distinctive in these terms.

- *Career history:* the breadth, depth and form of previous work experience—paid and unpaid—provided a clue to the skills and capabilities brought to the HCA role by the post holder, as well as giving an insight into future career intentions.

- *Motivations and aspirations:* HCA aspirations and motivations were viewed as likely to influence how individuals embraced their work role: what they sought from the role, whether and how they were keen to develop within it.

What form does the HCA role take?

A number of means were used to explore the structure and shape of the HCA role:

First we explored the HCA support-orientation. This involved exploring who the support worker actually assists, with three main candidates emerging in the case of the HCA: the nurse, the patient, and the ward team. Clearly the three are related and indeed potentially complementary: in supporting the patient by carrying out direct care tasks HCAs are supporting nurses by relieving them, and at the same time helping out the ward team. But it is an empirical question as to whether different actors place a particular emphasis on any one of these forms of support, with implications for how the HCA is viewed and treated.

Second we examined what constitute the 'good' HCA. Beyond formal job descriptions, different stakeholders—HCAs, nurses, ward managers, and patients—will have a view about what makes a 'good' HCA; the attitudes and behaviours they expect from the 'high performing' HCA.

Third we considered the tasks performed by HCAs. At the heart of exploring the form assumed by the HCA role are the activities undertaken by the post holder: their substantive character, the frequency with which they are undertaken, and their configuration within job boundaries. To facilitate a characterization of the role in these terms, tasks and activities were bundled under the following headings—these drew in part on the distinctions drawn at the outset of Chapter 1, although here they are refined:

- *Direct patient care:* tasks that address the patient's basic needs on the ward and involve direct physical contact of a non-technical or non-specialist nature: for example, bathing, feeding, and toileting.

- *Indirect patient care:* patient care that is not of a technical or specialist nature and does not involve physical contact. This includes making beds, serving meals or drinks, cleaning around the bedside, and assisting with patient-related paperwork such as admissions and theatre check lists.

- *Pastoral care:* providing general support to the patient or relative that is unrelated to patients' physical condition: for instance, reassuring patients or their relatives, helping confused patients, and dealing with the non-medical queries of patients.

- *Ward/team-centred:* tasks that are one step removed from direct patient care, usually occurring away from the bedside and in communal areas, including clerical or administrative tasks, answering the telephone, keeping stores stocked, attending handover sessions, and updating members of staff during the shift.

- *Technical/specialist care:* clinical/medical tasks and procedures that require dedicated training, such as monitoring and recording patient observations, dressings and wound care, electrocardiograms (ECGs), cannulation, catheter care, and taking blood samples.

A number of more specific themes related to the shape of the HCA role were explored. We examined the degree of differentiation and overlap between HCA and nurse activities: how far was the HCA extending its role to take on traditional nurse tasks? Consideration was given to where the core of the HCA role lay and what form any extension of the role took. Finally we were concerned with whether the tasks undertaken by post holders combined in different ways to produce different types of HCA.

What are the consequences of the HCA role for the three main stakeholders: HCAs themselves, nurses and patients?

We have seen that for each of the main stakeholders the HCA role has the potential to unleash both positive and negative outcomes. These outcomes are not necessarily mutually exclusive; they might conceivably coexist in tension, suggesting some ambiguity towards the HCA role.

For the HCA we considered the extent to which the role is a 'dead-end' or degraded, and whether it provided opportunities for development and enrichment. These outcomes were assessed by exploring:

- how HCAs were managed: how they were treated in terms of their grading, performance management, training, and voice;
- the treatment of HCAs by nurses and other actors at the ward level;
- HCA job satisfaction;
- what HCAs 'liked' and 'disliked' about the role;
- the emotional impact of the role on post holders.

For the nurse we considered if the HCA was of value, contributing meaningfully and effectively to their working lives or whether the role added new burdens and risks to be managed. These consequences were addressed by looking at:

- how nurses used HCAs and how they were perceived to contribute to nurse activities;
- whether nurses had any difficulties in dealing with and relating to HCAs, and if so what form these took.

Finally, we assessed the impact on the patient: whether the HCA role provided a less intimidating, more accessible form of care to that available from professional staff or whether it was a source of more diluted care. These outcomes were looked at by assessing:

- whether patients could tell the difference between HCAs and nurses;
- whether patients developed a different type of relationship with HCAs and nurses;
- and if so, what form this took and whether it mattered to patients.

Analytical framework

The analytical framework underpinning the pursuit of these questions comprised three main elements. The first was related to whether there were contingent influences on the nature and consequences of the HCA role. There are grounds for suggesting that as a nationally resourced and regulated service, the NHS encourages a basic standardization in service and work organization. Such standardization might be seen to foster similarities across the sector in terms of who is likely to take up the HCA role, what they do, and how it impacts. A more contingent view might hold that the HCA role is sensitive to a number of influences which produce variation in these respects. The contingent factors might plausibly include: the region, with local labour market factors affecting, for example, the supply of individuals into the unregulated nursing workforce; the Trust, with some residual control over the formulation and implementation of policies and practices as they relate to their workforce; and clinical area, the form and outcomes associated with the HCA role being dependent on the kind of patients, care tasks, and processes required in different sorts of clinical division.

The second element of the framework suggests an explanatory relationship between the key questions posed in this study. It might be argued that who HCAs are, in terms of their backgrounds, aspirations, and motivations, influences the form or shape of the role, which in turn impacts on its consequences for different stakeholders. Such a perspective places greater weight on individual agency within or overriding the institutional constraints set by the NHS, the Trust, or the division: the HCA role is seen as more malleable and sensitive to the capabilities and interests of those taking it up.

The third element is rooted in a stakeholder perspective. It is likely that HCAs, nurses, and patients come to the HCA role with some shared aims, perhaps related to the contribution of the role to care quality, but also some divergent interests, reflecting more specific group concerns and values. A stakeholder perspective encourages consideration of whether there is a consensus on the nature of the HCA role and its consequences, or whether the role has become a site of contestation, subject to pressures from stakeholders with competing identity-based aims.

Research methods

The research was mainly focused on four case study Trusts drawn from different parts of England—South, Midlands, North, and London. Originally the intention had been to focus on Trusts in the South, Midlands, and the North. As the research progressed it became clear that the distinctive nature of the London health economy required the inclusion of a London case study Trust. The same multi-methods approach was adopted in each case: this was designed to generate a detailed and comprehensive picture of the HCA role in two clinical areas—general medicine and general surgery—and one sensitive to the views of different stakeholders. The fieldwork was undertaken in three main phases covering a 30-month period: spring 2007 to autumn 2009.

Phase 1 (spring 2007 to late autumn 2007)

The initial phase took the form of semi-structured interviews with senior figures from Trusts beyond our core cases in the South, the Midlands, and the North regions. These interviews were designed to address our first research question on the strategic use of HCAs. They also provided the basis for the selection of our case studies. A small number of these regional Trust interviews were conducted on completion of the case study fieldwork as a means of calibrating the general case study findings. The intention was to interview the nursing director, human resources director, and nursing staff representative from either UNISON or the RCN across the three regions. During this phase a total of 37 individuals across nine Trusts, in addition to those carried out at our case study Trusts, were interviewed.

Phase 2 (late autumn 2007 to summer 2009)

This phase comprised intensive qualitative case study fieldwork in four Trusts, hereafter referred to as South, Midlands, North, and London. These Trusts were studied sequentially and in that order, with three months being devoted to each. Background details on the case study Trusts are presented in Table 3.1.

It can be seen that there was some variation in Trust structure, stage of development, and catchment area. In terms of structure, two of the Trusts—South and North—were quite large teaching hospitals, while the other two were traditional district general hospitals (DGHs). With the exception of Midlands, the Trusts had at least two sites, often at some distance from one another. Trusts were at slightly different stages of development. None had achieved Foundation Trust status but one, London, had submitted an application. As a consequence, London was the most financially robust of the Trusts. The others were less secure in these terms, Midlands, in particular, facing acute financial difficulties in the recent past, resulting in workforce reductions. There were some noteworthy differences in the socioeconomic locations of the Trusts: unemployment around Midlands was relatively high at 9 per cent, while the Midlands

Table 3.1 Case study sites

	South	**Midlands**	**North**	**London**
Sites	Multi	Single	Multi	Multi
Size	Medium teaching	Large DGH	Large teaching	Medium DGH
FT status	Preparing	Preparing	Preparing	Applied
Finance	Clawing back	Turnaround	Fragile	Surplus
Workforce adjustment	Controls	Reductions	Controls	None
Local area unemployment	7%	9%	6%	6%
Local area BME population	17%	24%	12%	26%

BME, black and minority ethnic; DGH, district general hospital; FT, Foundation Trust and London cases were located in areas of high ethnic diversity: in both catchment areas around a quarter of the local population was from black and minority ethnic (BME) groups.

The first Trust, South, completed during this phase was effectively a double case (see Table 3.2), in terms of the volume of work undertaken: two of the hospital's three sites were studied in considerable detail. This allowed for a testing and sharpening of the research tools. In each case study, three wards were selected from both the medical and surgical divisions, and although there was some variation in the precise patient mix between these wards across the different Trusts, they were similar enough in these terms to allow meaningful comparisons within and between case studies. The chosen wards typically included an emergency facility, a medical or surgical assessment unit, and where possible (in three of the four cases) wards on at least two Trust sites were included. A total of 29 wards across seven sites were covered in the research.

In each case the following qualitative research work was completed: interviews, observation, and focus groups.

Interviews

We aimed to conduct around 50 semi-structured interviews in each case study. This target was achieved in all cases; in three of the four it was significantly exceeded. Around a dozen senior managers (executive directors, divisional managers, and matrons) were interviewed per case to provide an overview of developments at the Trust and a corporate perspective on workforce issues. In each ward around six interviews were conducted covering three HCAs, a Band 5 and 6 nurse and the (Band 7) ward manager or senior sister (hereafter referred to as the ward manager). These interviews were wide-ranging, touching on all of the main themes covered in the research. Nurses and HCAs were asked to fill out a short pro forma, providing some structured information on their backgrounds. The interviewees were mainly selected by the ward

Table 3.2 Case study qualitative fieldwork

	South	Midlands	North	London	Total
Hospital sites	2	1	2	2	7
Wards	10	6	6	7	29
Staff interviews	96	62	50	65	273
Ward observation (hours)	111	60	51	53	275
Patients interviewed/focus groups	25	19	23	27	94

manager, but survey data (see later) indicate that in terms of background our HCA and nurse interviewees were generally similar to the wider population, suggesting that those interviewed were fairly representative of the ward HCA and nurse workforces. As Table 3.2 highlights, a total of 273 interviews were completed.

All interviews were digitally recorded and fully transcribed. These transcriptions were used in different ways. They were coded according to the main themes informing the study. There was also some processing of the transcription data. For example, an open question seeking life histories for HCAs was used to map and present structured career journeys. There was also some scope to quantify some of these data, plotting, for instance, the regularity with which HCAs 'liked' or 'disliked' aspects of their role.

Observation

Given that workers are not always able to clearly describe what they do at the workplace (Barley and Kunda, 2001), a programme of observation was undertaken. In each case, a medical and surgical ward was selected, and two HCAs plus a Band 5 or 6 nurse were observed for one early shift. A total of 275 hours of observation were completed on 11 wards. Observation took the form of non-participant shadowing of individual HCAs and nurses throughout an 'early shift'. The research team was also a common presence on the wards, attending ward and 'handover' meetings. Where possible, and to aid triangulation, those observed were members of staff who had previously been interviewed and consented to being shadowed. The observation data took two forms. First, there was a structured recording of what those observed were doing at each moment, where they were doing it, for how long, and which actors were involved. Addressing the comparative structure of HCA and nurse roles, observation data were analysed quantitatively according to the proportion of shift time spent on different activities and the length of time devoted to them. Second, field notes were taken during the shift in the form of direct quotes and reminders about incidents. These notes were expanded upon during observee 'down-time' and fully written up at the end of the shift before the researcher left the hospital.

These observation data were processed and used in a variety of ways. The field notes were coded according to key themes. Some discrete incidents and episodes, described in considerable detail, were drawn upon to illustrate and reinforce findings from other data sources. The field notes were also processed to map and pick up on patterns of activities. For example, they were used to plot differences in activity according to tasks between HCAs and nurses as well as between wards in different clinical areas.

Focus groups

Former patients were invited to participate in a series of focus groups at each Trust with the aim of gathering their views on the HCA role. These focus group sessions lasted between 90 minutes and two hours, with all sessions recorded. Almost 100 patients across the four case studies took part in these focus groups.

On the basis of all the qualitative data gathered, a full and substantial report was produced for each case study Trust. These reports were subject to feedback from and debate within the respective Trusts to guard against factual inaccuracies and any significant misinterpretation of events.

Phase 3 (spring 2009 to late autumn 2009)

The final phase of the research was devoted to generating quantitative survey data. The decision to conduct surveys only after the qualitative research phase, rather than before, was influenced partly by a desire to develop an understanding of, and a strong relationship with, each of the Trusts before embarking upon a substantial survey activity. More importantly, findings from the qualitative phase fed into the questionnaire development, guiding the surveys' focus and informing item construction. Three surveys were carried out in each Trust, covering HCAs, nurses, and patients. Response rates across all three surveys averaged 41 per cent for nurses and 51 per cent for HCAs and patients. In total, the surveys captured the views of 746 HCAs, 689 nurses, and 1651 former patients. A report with a full set of results along with extensive commentary and benchmarked analysis was produced each Trust. These again provided the basis for a discussion with the Trusts, and an opportunity to explore interpretations of the findings.

The surveys could not cover the wide range of issues dealt with during the qualitative phase of the study, so the focus was narrowed and sharpened. In the case of the HCA and nurse surveys, the aim, in part, was to gather descriptive data on aspects of our key themes: who HCAs and nurses were; what they did; and how the HCA role impacted on stakeholders.

The patient survey was focused on a number of basic issues, namely, whether patients could distinguish HCAs from other members of the ward team, and if they could, how they viewed them, especially relative to nurses.

The three research phases generated a rich and multifaceted database. In presenting the findings, the qualitative and quantitative material derived from the four case studies is used and combined in a flexible way, maximizing understanding and insight into any given theme: in some instances the qualitative material provides the initial context for the presentation of the more focused and structured survey data; in others, the survey data are presented upfront, the qualitative material being used to help explain the patterns revealed.

Key themes and narratives

In summary, this project explored the nature and consequences of the HCA role in secondary healthcare from a number of different perspectives. These are set out in Figure 3.1 and highlight the multi-case, the multi-divisional, the multi-methods, and the multi-stakeholder approach adopted to explore our research questions: who HCAs are, what they do, and how they have impacted.

These multiple perspectives provide the key themes and narratives for the presentation and discussion of the findings. The findings presented in the book revolve around what might be viewed as similarities and differences linked to these four dimensions:

- *Multi-case:* if the findings on the role and consequences of the HCA are similar across the four case study Trusts, it would suggest that there are some powerful sector-wide factors driving such standardization; if, however, differences emerge between the Trusts, it would hint at the influence of local factors on the role of the HCA linked perhaps to Trust conditions, policies, and practices.

- *Multi-division:* similarly, if the HCA role and its consequences are shared across general medical and general surgical wards, sector standardizing

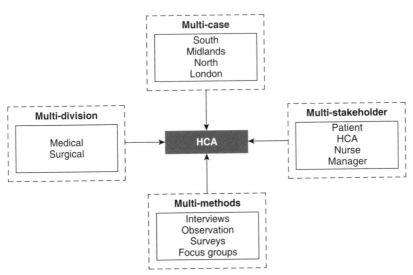

Figure 3.1 Multiple perspective approach.

forces would again seem to be at play; differences between these divisions would, however, suggest that the role is sensitive to clinical area, a function perhaps of different patient conditions generating distinctive routines and role requirements.

- *Multi-methods:* the application of different research techniques in a case study context, often referred to as triangulation (interviews, surveys, and observation) was designed to provide some confirmation of findings on the HCA role from contrasting methodological perspectives. The findings might, however, diverge, the source of such divergence perhaps lying in the nature of the research technique or in a genuine contradiction and ambiguity towards the HCA role.

- *Multi-stakeholder:* in seeking the views of different stakeholders—HCAs themselves, nurses, and patients—one outcome is a consensus between the groups on the nature and consequences of the HCA role. However, equally plausible is a variation in views between the stakeholder groups, suggesting that perspectives on the HCA role might be shaped by divergent group interests and values.

The book now turns to a presentation of the findings.

Chapter 4

Healthcare assistants as a strategic resource

> Senior manager_North: Support workers are an essential part of the nursing workforce but I think they are underdeveloped. As an organisation we haven't necessarily invested in their education and development to the extent that we perhaps could have done, and that might be one of the reasons why people haven't picked up on these roles to make a greater contribution.

If the healthcare assistant is to be used as a relief, substitute, apprentice, and co-producer, senior managers in Trusts explicitly need to consider the nature and deployment of the role in these terms. Trusts might be seen to strategically address the HCA role in various ways, reflecting a strong and a weak definition of the term 'strategic': a strong strategic approach indicates a clear attempt to link the role in a proactive way to the pursuit of broader Trust goals, say, related to care quality or patient access. A weak strategic approach suggests that the HCA role might well be considered at these senior management levels, but only in response to more immediate pressures or in a manner much less clearly related to wider Trust aims. A Trust might be seen to take a third, non-strategic, option, with the HCA simply not considered at all as an issue at senior management levels.

This chapter serves a number of purposes. First, by drawing on the interviews with 37 senior managers and union representatives across nine Trusts in three different regions—South, Midlands, and North—it provides a general picture of whether and how HCAs were viewed and deployed as a strategic resource. Second, the chapter explores the use of the HCA as a strategic resource in a more detailed way by focusing on our four case study Trusts. The value of concentrating on our four core cases in this way naturally lies in providing insight into how senior management viewed and used HCAs at Trust level. In addition, it gives some context to and backdrop for the main research findings as presented in the succeeding chapters.

The picture to emerge across all of the Trusts covered in this chapter as it relates to the strategic use of HCAs is a very similar one. It suggests that whilst typically valued as a resource, various constraints limited a strong strategic approach to the HCA role at senior management level. A weaker strategic approach finds some support, with HCAs periodically viewed and used by senior managers to address immediate needs and pressures. This is not to detract from some variation between the Trusts in the perception and the deployment of the role in these terms, a reflection of local conditions, organizational status and management style.

The chapter is divided into two main parts. The first is founded upon the 37 manager interviews in nine Trusts, considering the visibility and treatment of workforce matters at a senior management level, and then the planned use (or not) of HCAs as a relief, substitute, apprentice, and co-producer. The second part of the chapter provides a discussion on the strategic issues facing our four main case study Trusts, and how, if at all, these shaped their nursing workforce agenda and their treatment of the HCA role.

A regional picture

Workforce issues at corporate level

In considering the regional picture, attention focused on the general challenges facing the Trusts and whether and how these had filtered down to shape, in a general sense, workforce issues and, in particular, the management of HCAs. The main challenges facing the Trusts in the three regions were presented in terms of performance and finance. For those Trusts which had achieved Foundation Trust (FT) status, these challenges were somewhat less severe: after all, they had acquired their FT status on the basis of robustness in these terms. As noted by a manager in one, 'The last couple of years have been good to the Trust in terms of performance and finance'. But this was not necessarily the case; a manager in another Foundation Trust stressed that, 'the finances are a huge challenge at the moment'. The preoccupation with such matters often drove out workforce issues as a primary concern at senior management levels:

> Northern Trust: You wouldn't find them [workforce issues] explicitly as a heading. We have a Trust Board that's been dominated by parts of our strategic agenda.
> Midlands Trust: There is a business plan … But I wouldn't say there's much in there about workforce.

At the same time, workforce issues did emerge unprompted as a challenge in most of the regional Trusts, albeit mainly in a weak strategic form. First, workforce issues arose as a reaction to local labour market conditions. This was the case in a Northern Trust that was facing recruitment difficulties, especially amongst nurses. Second, such issues arose in the context of attempts to reduce headcount in response to financial pressures. As a Midlands Trust stressed:

> Midlands Trust: We committed to take seven hundred and fifty headcount out last year, but during the course of the year we took about half of that out … And balanced the rest with vacancy freezes etc.

Third, workforce issues were given prominence as Trusts sought to review skill mix, mainly in pursuit of cost efficiencies. This was apparent in a Southern Trust, where consideration of skills inevitably touched on support workers and their numbers relative to registered staff:

> Southern Trust: We've had a lot of discussion when the budget setting was being done this year to triangulate the establishment against the acuity and dependency tool that we were using and that led to a lot of discussion . . . The tool sort of tells you what your total establishment should be, but you then have to have discussions around skill mix.

In a related process, the reorganization of wards and the introduction of patient care pathways in a Midlands Trust led to a review of workforce number and skill mix:

> Midlands Trust: Because of the new orientation of the wards and layouts now, and also because of the patient pathways that are being revisited and reviewed, it's likely that we're going to need around five hundred whole-time equivalent extra support workers by the time the new hospital is fully operational.

There were examples of a stronger strategic approach to workforce issues, but these were much less common. In one instance, there was recognition of the link between workforce structure and broader organizational change:

> Northern Trust: We've got a bit of a dichotomy in terms of our capacity which we've always known would be around this time and that's in relation to continuing to manage an acute service whilst, at the same time, changing every element of that service ready to go in to the new hospitals. So we've got a very big organisational development plan which is seeking to influence attitudes, so that we don't move into beautiful new facilities with the same old approach to some things. And with that comes the change in the workforce.

In another more striking example, a Midlands Trust articulated a much stronger link between workforce issues and Trust well-being, reporting on this link regularly at Board level:

> Midlands Trust: At every single Board meeting there's an integrated performance report based on workforce aligned with clinical productivity and efficiency and also the operations and the finance of the organisation … I think they've made a conscious decision here … and that they felt because of the leadership issues, the quality issues,

and then the impact that that had on morale and the culture within the organisation, that workforce was a priority.

In short, general workforce issues remained downstream of matters related to performance and finance, only arising in the search for cost efficiencies or in the context of labour market pressures.

Policy goals and the HCA

In focusing more specifically on whether and how HCAs had been considered in strategic terms, it would be fair to say that amongst our regional Trusts the role did not figure with much prominence on the senior management agenda, either at Board or executive director level. This is not to deny the general value placed on HCAs by senior managers:

> Southern Trust: [HCAs are] invaluable, absolutely invaluable. I could take you to the ward that I was a ward sister of until three years ago and introduce you to some of the HCAs there who, you know, they are mentioned by patients in the thank you letters, they are acknowledged for the huge difference particularly in the psychological support to patients, more so in fact than some of the qualified nurses.

Indeed, there were exceptions to the neglect of the role at this level: the manager from a Northern Trust, considering workforce issues in the context of organizational change, goes on to note two important downstream changes:

> Northern Trust: One is the change in the pattern of healthcare, and therefore we will be wanting to use our healthcare support worker colleagues in a different way. And the second one is in relation to the affordability of the workforce for the future, which again drives potentially a change, so that we look to more Band 1 and Band 4 healthcare support worker colleagues.

There were, however, few instances of interviewees raising the development of the HCA role in an unprompted way, whether as a challenge or workforce issue facing the Trust. Even when prompted, the HCA role did not emerge as a major focus of senior management interest. When asked if the role entered discussions at this level, a manager in a Midlands Trust noted:

> Midlands Trust: On the Board, no. In the HR group and the workforce plans that get sent to the Health Authority, yes, but not in any great detail. That's the reason we've now appointed our workforce planning manager.

It was a view echoed in another Trust by a deputy chief nurse:

> Northern Trust: I wouldn't say they're regularly discussed [unregistered staff], I mean, but there is an HR element at every Board meeting where there's an HR report that talks about some of these elements in some detail. But there's a nursing report that goes to the Board, not as a nursing, the chief nurse takes other reports to the Board but we have had a workforce paper within the last year, but it's not something that goes

regularly as an active agenda item … I suppose when we talked about it last there was a real issue with nurse staffing within the organisation.

While not figuring prominently at senior management levels, attempts to use or to develop the role were highlighted. These can be related to the use of the role as a relief, substitute, and apprentice, although it was difficult to find any acknowledgement of the HCA as a co-producer. Again in the main such attempts displayed a weak rather than strong strategic orientation.

Relief

The role of the HCA as a relief, implicitly relieving the nurse of much of the direct and indirect patient care, came through in perceptions of the HCA role amongst senior managers across these Trusts:

> Northern Trust: They're [HCAs] the fundamental people that support the registered nurses to do that and support their role … So those people at care support level are very fundamental to providing our patient care, particularly with regards to nutrition and those types of things.

There was some acknowledgement of the growing importance of this role in the context of new performance measures related to the quality of care. If the HCA is increasingly accountable for direct and indirect care then the Trust's well-being becomes dependent on the delivery of these tasks:

> Midlands Trust: The contact between the patient and members of staff a lot of the time is with the healthcare support workers. So some of your quality measures could be dictated by the quality of care provided by those healthcare support workers. So if that's not taken seriously in terms of infection rates, and if you look at things like the [National Care Quality Commission] inpatient survey, a lot of those results could be dictated by the quality of care provided by the healthcare support workers, not so always your doctors and your qualified nurses.

In this Midlands Trust it was clear that the HCA role had been very much developed with these concerns in mind:

> Midlands Trust: We recognised that in the ward environments, some of the audits were undertaken by healthcare support workers on, 'are you washing your hands?', and actually they're the ones that are stopping doctors who are wearing wristwatches, saying 'don't wear that, do you understand you can bring infection in to this environment'. And they've been very much empowered to do that.

Substitute

It was, however, as a substitute that senior Trust management was most preoccupied with the HCA role. This interest assumed a number of forms. First, and as already implied, the greater use of HCAs relative to nurses figured prominently in the dilution of skill mix, with the explicit aim of reducing labour costs. This was stressed by a Trust manager in the Midlands:

> Midlands Trust: Some of the things we did last year in nursing was we changed the shift patterns and that allowed us to take seventeen nursing posts out by changing shift patterns. We balanced some of what we lost in terms of registered staff by introducing cheaper support worker type roles, so that allowed us to take the equivalent of posts out.

In the case of the former, Northern Trust, this cost saving was achieved through the use of Band 3 HCAs with an extended role rather Band 5 or 6 nurses. However, the employment of HCAs as a cost-efficient measure was also illustrated by their concentration in Band 2 posts. In almost all of the regional Trusts, the overwhelming proportion of HCAs was in Band 2; indeed in one Northern Foundation Trust, it was noted that Band 3 was hardly used at all:

> Northern Trust: We just have at the moment within our Trust, people that are Band 2 level care support workers and then we have our Band 5 registered nurses, and we've not got anything very much in between, if I'm really honest.

The scope available to Trusts to use the HCA in this way to dilute skill mix, so reducing labour costs, might be related to the easy availability of such workers in the local labour market: with the role unregulated, Trusts were able to impose extremely low barriers of entry into the role. Asked about entry criteria, a manager at a Southern Trust noted:

> Southern Trust: I haven't got anything specific … You know, for a Band 3 healthcare assistant an NVQ level 3 is desirable, for a Band 2 an NVQ level 2 is desirable. But it's really looking at the characteristics of the person.

It is unsurprising, therefore, that none of the regional Trusts had difficulty attracting a plentiful supply of applicants to the HCA role:

> Midlands Trust: We're always over, oversubscribed. Every time we advertise [for HCAs], inundated.

Second, a number of Trusts were seeking to use the support role as a substitute by developing Band 4 posts. Such an approach represents a form of dilution through the use of such Band 4 posts rather than registered nurse posts. As a manager at a Southern Trust noted:

> Southern Trust: We need to look at the skill mix in a different way, not just the sort of qualified/unqualified but a more three-way split with a middle ground of associate practitioner [Note: Typically a Band 4 post] … Or if it's not associate practitioner in the broad sense, is there something different.

It is therefore clear that support roles were being used as a form of substitution in pursuit of cost efficiencies in a couple of different ways: a predominantly Band 2 HCA workforce with few Band 3s reduced costs at the unregistered end of the nursing workforce, while the replacement of staff nurses with Band 4 support roles diluted and depressed costs at the registered–unregistered workforce interface.

Apprentice

The HCA role might be used in an apprenticeship capacity, both as a means of nurturing 'high performing' individuals within the HCA role and/or as a way of providing a future supply of 'grow your own' registered nurses. There were, however, few signs that Trusts had adopted a strong strategic approach to the HCA role in these terms through the development of supportive practices and systems. There were exceptions, most notably one of the Northern Trusts which had established a so-called 'apprenticeship model', seeking to establish clear career pathways allowing HCAs to move up and through the bands. The intention was to recruit a cohort of trainee HCAs, taking them through the different career levels:

> Northern Trust: We're aspiring to an apprentice healthcare assistant role and have developed a framework which has just been shared and will be rolled out across the Trust in the next couple of weeks subject to full approval by the clinical body, in regard to progression through Bands 1 through to Band 4 and then hopefully in to nurse education.

Elsewhere, HCA training and development were rooted mainly in NVQ accreditation, operating with varying degrees of efficiency and effectiveness. (At the time of the research NVGs were the main form of accreditation. They have since been replaced by the QCF.) A number of generic problems associated with NVQ training emerged, such as a shortage of NVQ assessors and individual HCAs finding it difficult to take time away from the ward to train:

> Southern Trust: It's [NVQ training] always been on offer, and NVQ level 3, but we haven't had the resources to allow all of our support workers to access it.

More indicative of the unplanned approach to such training was the mismatch between training opportunities and development of the HCA role. More specifically, the availability of such opportunities had outstripped the scope to use the acquired skills in the HCA role. This reflected a failure of workforce planning at senior, and perhaps lower, levels of management: HCA were developing capabilities often not required or used:

> Northern Trust: At the moment we do encourage staff to do an NVQ level 2 and level 3 training, I think our problem at the moment is the job role we're expecting them to do in the wards isn't requiring them to be at that level. What we need to do is look at the job roles … and bundle these in to something that requires them to be at a higher level for them.

In the case of a 'grow your own' approach to future registered nurses, Trusts had developed secondment schemes, allowing a small number of HCAs to embark on nurse training. These were beginning to wither, often for reasons beyond the Trust's control, a consequence of SHAs, for example, withdrawing funding for such schemes:

> Northern Trust: We've had a good record in terms of people taking up professional training places from support worker roles. And that's one of the reasons, we're disappointed really in terms of the loss of the sponsored places for nursing, for example, in that this allowed you to be seconded in to the nurse training post on an equivalent of your salary and not actually take a bursary, which in fact might be a two thousand pounds a year drop, which on those sort of salaries would be significant really.

Beyond secondment schemes there was little evidence to suggest that Trusts were evaluating the future demand and supply of registered nurses needed, and exploring the development of HCAs as a means of addressing any shortfall.

Main case studies

The picture presented from these interviews with Trust managers in different regions of the country finds a strong resonance in the strategic use of HCAs in our four main case study Trusts: South, Midlands, North, and London. There is, however, some value in taking these four respective cases in turn and considering the following in each: the general pressures faced by them; how these pressures impacted on workforce issues; and in particular how, if at all, they affected the strategic use of the nurse support role.

South

At the time of the research, South operated on three sites, and been established on this basis for the last ten years or so. As a Teaching Trust, it faced a major challenge in seeking to balance the provision of general hospital services for the local population, with the development of specialist services across a far broader catchment area, embracing neighbouring counties, and, in relation to some services, well beyond. These concerns were compounded by the considerable financial pressures faced by the Trust. It had a major overspend, a hangover from trying to improve performance and increase capacity, but in addition it had not fared well under new NHS funding arrangements.

Workforce issues were highlighted by some senior managers at the Trust as a major corporate issue, with particular difficulties faced in recruiting and retaining some staff. A strategy document noted:

> Local factors make it difficult to recruit nursing staff, healthcare professionals and clerical and administrative staff because of the high cost of living [in the area] and in particular high property prices and competition from employers in an area of very low unemployment.

The Trust also had a somewhat diffuse organizational culture with one of its sites, in particular, at some distance from the main one, and with its own history and identity. Indeed, despite a general concern about labour supply, recruitment and retention difficulties were markedly less intense at this 'arms length' site, drawing upon a very different, less tight labour market in an area of lower living costs.

In response to these general pressures, the Trust launched a strategic review in 2004. This revolved around the need to clarify the sort of services to be provided by the Trust: secondary and general hospital services; specialist and tertiary services provided across the region; distinctive services founded upon the expertise of its researchers and clinical practitioners; and platform services, supporting, and enabling. At first sight, limited consideration was given to workforce issues, beyond the general goal of being 'an employer of choice' and 'valuing and caring for our staff'. However, many of the 'constraining factors' confronting the Trust and raised in its strategic review were seen to relate to the workforce:

- recruitment difficulties, already highlighted in the context of a tight labour market;
- increasing workforce regulation, particularly professionals' working hours;
- increasing labour costs, which, in combination with limited local resources and national skill shortages, was encouraging the search for new ways of working. As the review document noted:

> We [the Trust] will need to examine how services can be delivered differently ... Making these changes will undoubtedly require new roles and different approach to teaching and education.

The approach adopted by the Trust to address these workforce constraints and issues was much less clear. It appeared that general workforce issues were often driven out by broader, more pressing financial considerations. As a senior manager noted:

> If you asked me where is the [Trust's] workforce plan, I'm not sure there is a very mature one, and I think a lot of things get pushed down when you focus purely on finance.

A similar point was made by another senior manager, stressing the difficulties faced in 'getting to grips' with workforce issues given other, more immediate, pressures:

> People talk about workforce planning and workforce issues but there is a tendency to feel they are such big issues that we don't really have much control over them ... I guess in reality workforce planning does seem to take place at the margins, at the

periphery, yet if I'm really honest it doesn't engage me because it is not immediate enough for me.

In such circumstance, workforce issues appeared to be treated by senior managers as part of a compliance agenda, which essentially narrowed them to conformance with a limited range of metrics associated with the achievement of nationally set targets. In plotting progress towards the objective of making the Trust 'an employer of choice', the Trust's 2006/2007 Plan simply referred the reader to 'a balanced scorecard of performance indicators'. These included lowering vacancy levels, reducing sickness and turnover rates, controlling expenditure of agency staff, ensuring that 50% of staff fulfilled the mandatory training requirements, and 50% of non-consultant staff had completed their appraisals. Similarly, while the Trust's human resource strategy, formulated to cover the 2007–2010 period, noted an intention for 'the re-design and extension of roles to drive the HR agenda', it was difficult to uncover an action plan to progress such an agenda.

This pattern of broadly drawn workforce aspirations, driven off the strategic agenda by more pressing concerns, and narrowed to compliance with a few performance targets, was reflected in the Trust's approach to HCAs. The strategic review made specific mention of developing the HCA, noting the Trust 'must take account of pressures and opportunities to increase the role of the HCA'. This was echoed in the views of some senior managers at the Trust, stressing the growing significance of HCAs as the role of the nurse in the delivery of direct patient care weakened:

> Healthcare assistants have been pretty essential at the point at which nursing staff no longer see their primary role as washing and feeding and caring for patients.
>
> I see having support workers as a really important part of the workforce. … the practice nurse, the person that's registered, needs to do the assessment and the evaluation, but everything else in between can be done by an HCA.

The perceived importance of the HCA to healthcare delivery was not, however, reflected in any apparent consideration of the role at senior management levels. In March 2007, there were 672 whole-time equivalents (WTE), with 987 actual staff in post. This figure represented a noteworthy proportion of the Trust's total workforce, around 10% on a headcount and WTE measure. At the same time, the HCA workforce had been run down over recent years. Indicative of an HR agenda driven by immediate financial concerns, the Trust had been operating a recruitment freeze, in large part accounting for this drop. Although the Trust had also introduced a Band 3 ward housekeeper role, with one per ward, working a nine to five, Monday to Friday week, it was unlikely that the emergence of such a role would significantly impact on the need for HCAs.

Certainly it is difficult to conclude that the reduction in the number of HCAs reflected a more strategic consideration of the Trust's nursing workforce—an attempt to enrich the skill mix or to develop new roles in pursuit of new forms of service delivery—with HCAs rarely if ever, figuring in senior management deliberations. As a senior manager noted:

> I think they [HCAs] are a group which is managed and thought about at a lower level; I don't think we've ever talked about HCAs specifically ... We do review skill mix with a ratio of trained to untrained and we've just done another exercise, or the nursing directorate, have, and we're probably hoping to look at it again, so it's there in the kind of things we think about but we probably think about it in terms of saving money more than anything else.

Similar views were voiced by another senior manager:

> I think any decision about what we are going to do with HCAs is very arbitrary. I don't think they [the Trust Board] relate that at the moment to any business objectives

Midlands

The Midlands Trust had recently been through a significant organizational change, primarily forced by its status as a 'failing Trust'. This failure was mainly reflected in the Trust's financial state, but also in relatively poor performance against key national targets. The turnaround was driven by a new Chief Executive and recently appointed directors in key executive positions. At the core of this turnaround was a three-year financial recovery plan designed to address a significant financial deficit. The change programme had to confront a strong organizational culture, which, from a management perspective, had some strengths but also created certain difficulties.

Based on a single site, and one of the main sources of employment in the city, the Trust had attracted a close knit and stable workforce. It was noted that 'everybody knew everybody' in the Trust, and there were even family connections within the workforce, relatives often working alongside one another or in different parts of the organization. In combination these characteristics generated a strong commitment to the Trust:

> On the whole people are quite passionate about working in [the Trust] ... There is a genuine passion for the Trust amongst some employees.

At the same time, however, this very culture was seen by some to have contributed to the Trust's past difficulties particularly its lack of financial control:

> [The Trust] was a really lovely place to work in but from a finance viewpoint there was really no control ... From a management point of view I just couldn't believe what I could have done if I'd wanted and nobody questioned it at all.

Indeed, despite, or perhaps because of this close knit culture, the Trust had a history of highly adversarial industrial relations:

> Industrial relations were a huge issue here … It was real, old banging of table, walking out of rooms.

This impression of an organization generating considerable loyalty but perhaps somewhat 'stuck in its ways' was reflected in its treatment and view of HCAs. It is noteworthy, for example, that the role's title at the Trust, nursing auxiliary, harked back to the original and longstanding Whitely grade label. It was a role supported by a hostess grade at Band 1 and in some wards by a similarly banded ward assistant role, both responsible for some basic cleaning and the provision of food to the patients.

The new management team's change programme seeking to address the Trust's financial difficulties, and some of these traditional organizational features, comprised various initiatives. There was, for example, an organizational redesign, which lead to a streamlining of the divisional structure. A number of these initiatives, however, focused on the workforce, often with a view to controlling or reducing labour costs. First, there was an attempt to move industrial relations away from its historical adversarialism to what management viewed as a 'partnership model'. This was seen as founded upon a more direct contact between management and the workforce, with the unions supporting rather than mediating this relationship. As the Trust's HR strategy noted:

> It is recognised that we need to do more to communicate and engage directly with staff … Direct communication with staff needs to be emphasised as the primary relationship, with the trade union interface being seen as supporting not driving.

Second, the Trust implemented a programme of workforce reductions: between 2006 and 2008, a total of 450 Trust jobs were lost. These losses were mainly achieved through natural wastage, with only 14 compulsory redundancies. Nonetheless, these reductions inevitably reduced workforce capacity and in so doing generated new service delivery pressures. These pressures were intensified by a third workforce development, a skill mix review. This review established a 70/30 skill mix across the Trust, based on a new template for ward staffing. The effect of the new template was a need to reduce the number of Band 6 registered nurses and Band 3 HCAs in post, relatively high-cost posts compared to nurse Band 5s and HCA Band 2s. The process effectively led to the downgrading of a not insignificant number of staff at these levels.

The outcomes of the Trust's change programme might be viewed in various ways. In terms of 'hard' outcome measures, there were some significant 'gains': patient satisfaction rates increased to the highest in the region and there was a dramatic reduction in the hospital-acquired infection rate, recognized by an award to the Trust. In general, industrial relations were perceived as less conflictual. As a senior manager noted:

> Trade unions work much closer with management and nursing and other professionals to actually see the big picture rather than obstructing all the time.

There had also been a perceived shift in senior management style, albeit with views differing on the nature of this change and its consequences. For some it was viewed positively as a much tighter, more focused and coherent style:

> The management style … is much more disciplined and robust and the formalities of whichever element you're looking at are managed much better.

For others the style had placed middle and junior mangers under considerable pressure. As one middle manager noted:

> I feel my colleagues, my peers, they've had a real battering and everyone is very, very nervous about their jobs; they don't want to put their heads above the parapet.

Indeed, this 'fear' was seen by some as pervasive. As one manager noted in referring to the regular open forums session where executive directors addressed all staff groups:

> When they've [the executives] finished and they say have you got any questions – no questions . . . and I think more and more now it's fear … I think it [the forum] should be a safe haven and it isn't.

On a broader scale, there were some in the Trust who felt the morale of frontline staff had also been weakened by the change programme:

> There's been a huge culture change because of the way that they manage and because of the financial situation that we have faced over the last three or four years; that's made life in the Trust difficult for a lot of people: particularly frontline staff because to them they're delivering the services; they don't necessarily see everything that goes on behind the scenes in terms of what we have to deliver from a financial point of view, all they see is that we're cutting costs and cutting posts.

North

The North case study Trust was established some ten years ago with the merger of three separate hospitals. Subsequently North became a somewhat sprawling organization acquiring a number of additional sites. Indeed partly as a consequence the Trust had found it difficult to develop a tight organizational culture and a clear, integrated identity. As a senior manager at the Trust noted:

> I'd struggle to define the [Trust's] culture; I could have a crack at defining the management culture, but whether there's something common to the way all of the clinical teams operate is more difficult to put your finger on.

In general, the Trust might be characterized as emerging from a period of uncertainty in terms of focus and financial well-being, but had still to fully establish itself on a stable or sustainable basis. This characterization was encapsulated by the Trust's position (at the time of the research) in relation to Foundation Trust status. Past weaknesses in meeting certain performance standards had delayed the application process, with any submission being unlikely in the next year or so.

In the recent past, the Trust had faced financial pressures and found it difficult to meet national performance targets. As a senior manager stated:

> We also went through a period about three years ago when we were under severe financial pressure ... The sort of 'million dollar question' is why we weren't able to crack [the financial] problems sooner. And it's quite a conundrum actually. It has been a big issue [at the Trust] for a long time.

These pressures had prompted various Trust responses, often focusing upon the workforce. One of the most significant was a recent de facto freeze on recruitment in 2007, which through natural wastage took around 650 employees out of establishment levels. It was, however, a fairly unplanned, opportunistic approach to workforce reduction, which had contributed to some weakening of staff morale. As one senior manager noted:

> Generally the vacancy freeze ... was seen to be negative across the organisation ... Nothing could compromise patient safety, these types of things, and it was expected that people would be redeployed or moved from one part of the Trust to the other, That was done with varying degrees of success: in some areas that happened but I certainly attended a number of discussions with staff side representatives where it was felt that certain groups were feeling the brunt more than others.

At the time of the research, there were signs that the Trust was moving onto a more even financial 'keel', prompting a renewed determination to address issues associated with managerial capacity, the better achievement of access targets, and the improvement of patient choice.

These strategic concerns found a faint 'echo' in the search for new work roles and ways of working. The Trust's recently published Nurse and Midwifery Strategy provided a dedicated section on 'Nursing and Midwifery Roles', with considerable emphasis placed not only on ways of working, but on the 'development of new roles'. However, Trust statements on new roles and ways of working remained vague, largely aspirational, and mainly focused on registered nurses rather than on HCAs. As a matron noted:

> In the nursing strategy there is something about modernising the workforce but I can't honestly say a big piece of work is being undertaken.

This is not to detract from isolated attempts by the Trust to develop nurse support role. There was some interest in developing Band 4 assistant practitioner roles in particular clinical areas. For example, there were ongoing attempts to train an advanced perioperative assistant within theatres to help registered nurses by performing the scrub role or assisting during recovery. The Trust had also taken up the housekeeper role, establishing it within wards as a Band 1 post. However, it was difficult to discern any meaningful senior management consideration of HCAs as a strategic resource within the Trust. As one senior manger stressed:

> Within the organisation at the moment we have very few examples of where we've moved away from a Band 2 role, whether people call that a healthcare assistant or a nursing assistant. I don't think yet we have got our approach to that sorted out. I don't think we've got a long term plan of where we're going to go with that. It's meant more piecemeal development where people have had a particular local enthusiasm for developing the role of support workers in a different way.

London

Established as a single site NHS Trust around 20 years ago, London assumed its present form when it merged with another single-site Trust, some half a dozen miles away, in the early 1990s. There was a considerable asymmetry in the size and range of services provided on the Trust's two sites, with the main site being by far the larger and more clinically diverse. Indeed, with different sites and their distinctive histories, it remained somewhat questionable whether the Trust had been able to develop a fully integrated culture.

Notwithstanding this divide, there was considerable consensus on the prevailing culture on the main site. This site was compact, facilitating the development of a fairly 'open' and 'friendly' organizational culture. This openness was symbolically expressed by the accessibility of the Trust Chief Executive and the directors, their office being located on the ground floor central corridor of the main site building:

> It's [the Trust] got a very open door culture. The board members are accessible to people … It's like [the chief executive's] office everyone knows where it is; there's nothing that stops anyone going and knocking on his door.

It was also a culture which quite heavily drew upon the local community, situated in outer rather than inner London, most of the staff living and commuting from within the Trust's catchment area.

The Trust had made considerable progress in seeking to become a Foundation Trust, submitting an application. As a Foundation Trust applicant, the organization was in sound financial health: the Secretary of State needs to classify a Trust in 'good order' in financial (and other terms) before that Trust can make an application. Between 2006–2009, London Trust had managed to generate a considerable financial surplus. The relative financial well-being of the Trust should not, however, detract from the challenges it faced.

One of the most pressing was the aging nature of the estate: there was an urgent need to maintain and update the main Trust buildings. Other challenges derived from the Trust's location. As a London Trust, it was facing some uncertainty over the continuity and development of certain services; plans were being formulated to reconfigure services in the capital. Partly related to its location on the outskirts of London, the Trust also faced quite intense competitive pressures for the provision of acute care services. There were a number of other Trusts in adjacent county areas, as well as Trusts within other parts of London providing such services. The Trust's search for competitiveness in these circumstances added to the importance of meeting national performance targets, and although the Trust was achieving in these terms, its rate for hospital-acquired infection remained relatively high.

With varying degrees of directness, these Trust challenges and issues found their way on to the workforce agenda. Located in outer London, the Trust had been operating with relatively high vacancy levels, the recruitment and retention of nurses, in particular, proving difficult:

> It's [nurse recruitment] a London issue. The problem for us is you've got London Trusts where they get more money because there's the inner supplement. We're right on the border so they only get the outer London supplement.

Skill mix was subject to a review, designed to fine tune the balance between efficiency and patient safety rather than to seek cost savings in response to financial pressures. There had been some past sensitivity to the skill mix issue, the Trust retreating from a headline 50/50 skills mix in its nursing strategy to 60/40. However, the major disruption for staff came less from any skill mix review and more from Trust moves towards a system of e-rostering. Introduced in 2008, e-rostering was seen not only as a means of reducing the time spent by ward managers on rostering, but as a way of standardizing shift patterns and reducing idiosyncratic forms of working that had emerged over the years. As one manager noted:

> E-rostering caused a right hullabaloo because it manages requests for shifts and [annual] leave a lot more stringently than the ward sisters were doing.

The impact of broader Trust concerns on ways of working, and, in particular, on the use and management of HCAs at the Trust was limited. In 2007, London Trust employed 361 HCAs, around half the number of nurses employed and constituting around 15 per cent of the total workforce. The Trust's senior managers placed considerable value on the HCA role. As one senior manger noted:

> I see complainants usually when something horrible has happened and somebody has died and they [relatives and friends] always point to staff who they think show that care and compassion, a high correlation with them being HCAs.

This appreciation of the HCA role encouraged the development of new nurse support roles. For example, a new Band 3 emergency room technician role, taking tasks off the registered nurse, was being created in the Trust. This was, however, a relatively isolated instance. Indeed the Trust's senior managers suggested there was considerable scope for further, more innovative use of HCAs:

> Having observed the HCA role as it has evolved, I think we've sometimes been a bit slow to recognise what their role really is and what they could contribute.

This was echoed in the views of a Trust middle manager:

> I still think that a lot of senior members of staff view HCAs as the ones that run in there to wash the patients and empty the bedpans … They don't realise HCAs can take on extra skills.

In short, therefore, London was a Trust not without challenges. These were in large part linked to its position on the fringes of the capital and fed through into workforce concerns, particularly associated with recruitment and retention. But the Trust's relative well-being had removed the urgency to address issues of workforce size and structure. This had an 'upside': workforce numbers were stable and punitive skill reviews absent. But London had not taken the opportunity to use this stability to explore the more innovative development of roles, not least amongst HCAs.

Summary

The purpose of this chapter was to consider whether and in what sense HCAs have been viewed and used by senior Trust managers as a strategic resource. If the HCA role was to be deployed in pursuit of a range of public policy goals, at the very least Trusts needed to display some interest in and engagement with the role at senior decision-making levels. The chapter explored these issues in two parts. The first drew upon interviews with senior managers in nine Trusts in different English regions, explicitly focusing on whether HCAs were regarded as a relief, a substitute, an apprentice, or a co-producer. The second focused on our four, core, Trust case studies, more generally assessing the challenges faced by these organizations, as well as whether and how these challenges had filtered down to shape the nursing workforce agenda, and particularly the treatment of the HCA role. The narrative emerging from both data sources presents a very similar picture. In the strongest sense of the term, the HCA had rarely been viewed strategically. In a weaker sense, the role had figured in ad hoc, opportunistic responses to immediate pressures. In the main, however, HCAs had not assumed prominence in senior management deliberations, casting doubt on their use as a strategic resource.

It might, with some legitimacy, be claimed that in general terms few, if any, occupational group in any employment context emerges at the heart of senior management discussion and decision-making. However, even leaving aside the weight placed upon the HCA role by national policy as outlined in Chapter 2, many of the individual Trusts covered in this chapter made explicit formal reference to using and developing the HCA role. In other words, Trusts were often trialling the HCA as a potential strategic resource, and less formally many of our respondents were highlighting the value they placed on the role. It is against the backdrop of this rhetoric extolling the HCAs' value that the lack of serious engagement by senior managers with the role becomes particularly noteworthy.

In certain instances, Trusts were seeking to develop the HCA role, linking it to the achievement of broader organizational objectives, associated, say, with improving care quality. In one Trust a new emergency room technician role was being introduced, whilst more generally, there was some interest in developing new Band 4 assistant practitioner roles. These instances, however, were rare. More typically, a Trust's workforce agenda was being driven by immediate financial and performance pressures, encouraging an interest in reducing labour costs. HCAs were often viewed and treated against the backdrop of this cost minimization agenda, with reviews seeking to dilute skill mix, or in some cases, to reduce workforce size.

At the same time, differences in the broad challenges facing particular Trusts, and how these might affect approaches to the development and management of the HCA role should not be overlooked. More specifically, in terms of pressures faced, our four case study Trusts were positioned in slightly different ways. As teaching hospitals, South and North were grappling with the provision of an array of general and specialist services across sprawling estates infrastructure. They were struggling to establish an integrated and coherent organizational identity, at the same time emerging from the legacy of financial and service underperformance, which had prompted workforce reductions. Midlands had been forced to address even more intense financial and performance pressures, implementing a turnaround programme based upon punitive measures in the shape of a major workforce downsizing and a cost-driven skill mix review. Only London appeared to be on even financial and performance keel, although located on the outskirts of the capital it still faced competitive and labour market challenges. Such differences between the Trusts provide an important context to the presentation of the more detailed findings set out in the succeeding chapters on the nature and consequences of HCA roles, findings which dig beneath senior management perceptions to explore how in practice HCAs were used and managed in our four Trusts.

Issues for reflection

The findings in this chapter suggest the need for senior Trust managers to consider:

- The relationship between the HCA role and the pursuit of broader corporate objectives.
- The development of an organizational infrastructure which promotes and supports the development of HCAs as a strategic resource.
- The development of a more consistent, coherent and transparent Trust approach to the use of HCAs.
- The recruitment and development of HCAs within the context of workforce planning systems for the nursing workforce.
- Optimizing the distinctive contribution made by HCAs to care quality.

Chapter 5

Backgrounds of healthcare assistants

> HCA_South: I've always wanted to do nursing, wanted to do the enrolled nursing, but ... as they've phased enrolled nursing out and then you have to have five GCSEs and sometimes even more than that to go to do nursing course, and I never had it ... so I thought the next best thing was becoming a healthcare assistant. HCA_Midlands: Looked after my mum really at home ... if I can do it for my mum I can do it for everybody else.

Introduction

This chapter explores the kinds of people attracted to the HCA role. More specifically, it considers the background of those taking up the post in terms of their: personal characteristics; work and life experiences; motivations and aspirations. A focus on HCA backgrounds has value in a number of different respects:

- First, there is a limited research literature on what might be termed 'atypical careers'; in other words, the careers pursued by those often on the margins of the labour market, commonly women with domestic responsibilities, sometimes from ethnic minority groups, and typically from lower economic classes. This study provides an opportunity to explore whether the HCA role attracts this type of individual and, if so, to assess their personal journeys to and within the role.

- Second, HCA backgrounds, particularly relative to those of the registered nurse, are crucial to establishing the identity of HCAs as an occupational group: HCAs might, in part, be defined by whether and how they differ from registered nurses in terms of their backgrounds.

- Third, the HCAs' backgrounds might, in turn, be linked to performance within the role. It will be recalled that public policymakers have presented the HCA as making a distinctive contribution to healthcare delivery. It is a contribution sometimes seen to lie in the tacit skills they bring to the role from their broader life experiences. More prosaically, HCA capabilities and skills which derive from their earlier career histories are likely to influence the efficiency and effectiveness with which they perform in the role.

- Fourth, the HCAs' personal circumstances—their domestic responsibilities, other interests and priorities, levels of household income, and individual aspirations—might well affect the post holder's general orientation to, and engagement with, the role. For example, such circumstance might relate to whether the HCA: 'crafts' the role; uses it as the basis for further career development; or draws upon it in a more transactional way.

- Fifth, a focus on backgrounds provides insight into the nature and the operation of the labour market for HCAs. As an unregulated role, there are few formal rules, constraints, or routines structuring the demand for and supply of HCAs. This generates uncertainty as to how the labour market for these workers functions: whether, for example, there are any discernible patterns in the kinds of people attracted to the role or in the de facto entry criteria used by trusts.

- Finally, unpacking HCA backgrounds represents a way of establishing a more meaningful, perhaps empathic, link to those performing the role. A mapping of life and work journeys is likely to provide a rich insight into those undertaking any work role, deepening an appreciation of the efforts they have made and the difficulties they have had to overcome. In the case of HCAs, this mapping is particularly important to an understanding of post holders given the limited information available on their backgrounds.

The chapter argues that the backgrounds of those taking up and performing the HCA role are likely to be determined by the interaction of demand and supply side factors. The background profile of HCAs is likely in the first instance to be driven by what Trusts demand in terms of numbers, capabilities, and personal qualities. These requirements are typically embedded in Trust staffing or establishment levels, in formal job descriptions, person specifications, and in the managerial practice of those with responsibility for HCA recruitment. Who HCAs are also relates to the local labour market supply: the types of individual likely to respond to Trust demand in terms of personal characteristics, past work experience, motivation, and aspirations.

The chapter is divided into two main parts: the first considers demand side requirements as they relate to HCAs and the second explores supply side responses.

The demand side

Trust requirements

Staffing requirements are related to skill mix: the balance between registered and unregistered nursing staff. While skill mix varied within our case study Trusts according to ward size and clinical area, all four Trusts had a 'headline' skill mix ratio: three Trusts claimed a 70/30 registered/unregistered staff split, the other suggesting a 60/40 ratio. Yet despite these headline figures, skill mix remained a lively policy space for senior management action.

The skill mix formula in Trusts was based on and reflected historical data crudely linking staff numbers to ward size, which had often been overtaken by organizational changes. This skill mix 'decay' or 'creep' had led to anomalies in the distribution of staff between divisions and wards, encouraging general attempts to sharpen such ratios, particularly by relating them more precisely to patient dependency and acuity. At the same time, the urgency of such attempts varied, largely reflecting the financial pressures faced by the Trust. It has been noted that in London, with its relatively sound financial situation, skill mix remained a low key issue; by contrast, in Midlands, a Trust involved in a major financial turnaround, skill mix had recently been used more aggressively by management to seek savings. This change was pursued not through a straightforward dilution of skill mix, but through the imposition of a shared staff template across the whole of the Trust, so removing resourcing idiosyncrasies between wards and divisions, and, specifically in the case of HCAs, reducing the number of Band 3 posts relative to Band 2.

At ward level, assumptions about skill mix ratios were enshrined in establishment levels, specifying in FTE terms, precise numbers of HCAs and registered nurses. These were crucial in determining the staff budget, typically devolved to the ward manager. While fixing the total funds available for ward staffing, the budget provided a degree of residual discretion to the ward manager to vary numbers employed on different grades. Although this discretion was not often used in any Trust, requiring approval by the matron or divisional manager at an even higher level, there were instances of attempts to change skill mix. For example, a ward manager in an emergency unit in London, sensitive to the high incidence of IV medication in her clinical area, was seeking to use the funds available for HCAs to employ more Band 5 nurses:

> Ward manager_London: I've got three Band 2s at the moment but they were actually here when I arrived, so I've kept them. They're excellent, but I want to change another two of my Bands 2s to make another Band 5 ... The majority of patients that come through here are medical and on admission they need IV antibiotics, IV fluids and a lot of intervention ... Unfortunately my Band 2s can't do the majority of work which does consist of the drugs, antibiotics plus IV fluids.

Comparing skill mix between the Trusts is a difficult task given differences in ward size and patient mix. In trying to control for these differences, a general comparison across the medical divisions can be made between those wards in three of the Trusts which comprised stroke patients. It can be seen in Table 5.1 that staff numbers per shift and the skill mix ratios were fairly similar, although it is noteworthy that in contrast to South and Midlands, London had more HCAs working the early shift than registered nurses.

In the case of four broadly comparable surgical wards across our four Trusts, the skill mix ratios are again not greatly out of line with each other (Table 5.2). In general, it is noteworthy that skill mix is richer for surgical than medical wards. However, the Midlands surgical ward has a slightly richer skill mix than in the other three Trusts: although on the early and late shifts this richness was

Table 5.1 Skill mix ratio on stroke wards (registered/unregistered staff)

	South	Midlands	North	London
Beds	23	15	n/a	22
Early	2/3	3/2	n/a	2/3
Late	2/2	2/1	n/a	2/2
Night	2/1	2/1	n/a	2/1

Table 5.2 Surgical ward skill mix ratio (registered/unregistered staff)

	South	Midlands	North	London
Beds	25	28	30	30
Early	4/2	4/1	4/2	4/3
Late	2/2	4/1	4/1	4/2
Night	2/1	3/0	2/1	2/2

mainly achieved by having one less HCA on shift than elsewhere, a reflection perhaps of the fact that Midlands was the Trust which had undergone the programme of workforce reduction and a major skill mix review.

The number of HCAs on a ward establishment needed to achieve these shift staffing ratios varied quite considerably, both within and between Trusts. As already implied, this was partly associated with clinical divisions and the related richness of the skill mix; for example, in Midlands where our ward level data are most reliable, five HCAs in total were employed on the general medical wards compared to nine on the general surgical wards.

The demand for HCAs was not, however, solely dependent on establishment levels and skill mix ratios. Many of the wards across all Trusts had HCA vacancies: of the 13 wards covered in London and the North, 11 had vacancies. Indeed vacancies of between a third and a half of the total HCA complement were not uncommon on a given ward. These vacancies were rarely a consequence of external local labour market shortages (see later in this chapter) but more often reflected HCA turnover and the lag which resulted in recruiting replacements. Such vacancies typically led to the use of bank or agency HCAs or, if not addressed in this way, to staffing pressures on any given shift. At the same time in the context of recruitment freezes, recently implemented in three of our Trusts, these vacancies could give rise to concerns about the adequacy of staffing levels and the quality of service provision. Such concerns were particularly apparent at Midlands, making the sharpest workforce reductions. As a Trust manager noted:

> Senior manager_Midlands: We haven't been able to advertise vacancies because we have to wait for the skill mix review outcomes … So areas like the stroke unit have been running with eight vacancies and it's affected the introduction of the new thrombolysis service, so it really has had a huge impact.

Much less attention had been devoted by Trusts to grade mix in seeking to shape their demand for HCAs. While Trusts had available two HCA bands plus an assistant practitioner level, reflecting an assumed variance in the size and nature of roles, there had been considerable reliance of Band 2 posts alone (see later section) and a marked reluctance to untangle how Band 2 and 3 roles might be differentiated and used within the ward to enhance care delivery. As a consequence, in the main, Trusts were seeking individuals to fill Band 2 roles:

> Senior manager_North: Within the organisation at the moment we have very few examples where we have moved away from Band 2 roles … We have started to get a small number of areas where they have developed different support roles, so perhaps Band 3 support workers, but they're in a minority. I don't think we have got our approach to that sorted out.

Recruitment

In all Trusts, the recruitment of HCAs was underpinned by corporate systems related to the advertisement of posts and the sorting out of the final details associated with an appointment. These systems were utilized and impacted in slightly different ways in the various Trusts. The HCA survey indicated (see Table 5.3) some noteworthy variation between Trusts in how applicants found out about vacancies. The main source of information about advertised posts was the Trust or NHS website, with around half hearing about the job from this source. A not insignificant minority of HCAs, close to a quarter, learnt about vacancies from a friend or relative. However, websites were a particularly common source of information in North and London. Perhaps unsurprisingly given the compactness of the site and close-knit character of the organizational culture, word of mouth was more prevalent at Midlands. In North the local press remained ineffective or not utilized as a form of communication.

There were also some Trust differences in the tightness of entry criteria to the role, which might have been more directly linked to local labour market conditions. Although in the main the Trusts did not have difficulty attracting applicants to HCA posts, Midlands was located in an area with relatively high unemployment (see Table 3.1) and could be more discriminating in its selection. It had instituted a tightly structured and in-depth schedule for interviews to HCA posts, designed to explore past work experience:

> Ward manager_Midlands: You sometimes get people who are in nursing homes but want to work more in an acute setting, but dependent on how many jobs we've got and where they've worked, we can be a bit more selective.

Beyond formal advertisement for the role and sorting out the final contract details, the recruitment of HCAs in all Trusts remained a ward-level process. While there were generic and broadly-drawn Trust job descriptions and person specifications for HCAs at Bands 2 and 3, these were often fine-tuned to reflect local ward needs, and the shortlisting and interviewing were all

Table 5.3 How HCAs heard about their current job (%)

	South	Midlands	North	London	p-value
A friend or relative	29	34	24	21	
Local press	21	16	9	21	$\chi^2 = 20.80$, $p = 0.014$
Trust/NHS website	46	47	60	58	
Job centre	4	4	7	1	

conducted by senior ward staff. Indeed there were instances of innovative practice, as in the case of a ward in London where a HCA was a member of the interview panel.

More significantly, a broadly-drawn job and person specification applied at ward level, left considerable discretion for ward managers to interpret and informally apply requisite entry qualifications. For example, at London, which had formally stated a preference for applicants with NVQ level 2, many individuals were taken on without such a qualification in the expectation that this would be acquired whilst working at the Trust. This opened the way for a range of less formal, more impressionistic criteria to be used by those assessing applicants:

> Ward manager_London: The last lot [of HCAs] … we were looking for experienced people, however we took an applicant who's come from Woolworths – never done care work before but interviewed very well, although she had no hospital experience or care experience, she had qualities in different ways. She had customer care, she was empathetic, and we took her and she's doing absolutely wonderful.

There were frustrations associated with the recruitment process, particularly amongst ward managers. With responsibility for placing the advertisement and then finalizing the contract of employment often lying at corporate level, ward managers expressed some dismay at the slow pace of developments associated with the processing of the paperwork:

> Ward manager_North: [HCA recruitment is] fairly bureaucratic and the people that support this process in terms of putting ads out, setting up interviews, doing all the processing of the work are really poorly paid. Only yesterday I was chasing round to get the right number on the right bloody request form for the job to find the right person so that we can carry on. So it's just hard work.

There were also concerns about the numbers of potential HCAs turning up for interview once shortlisted: managers had to formulate a shortlist on the assumption that many of those asked for interview would simply not show up:

> Ward manager_London: This time we had seventy applications for two posts, I shortlisted twenty and I had ten turn up.

The supply side

In general, there was a plentiful supply of applicants for HCA posts across all four Trusts. Ward managers and others consistently noted the large numbers responding to advertised HCA posts:

> Matron_Midlands: It seems to be fairly easy [to recruit HCAs] and the feedback I get from my [Band] 7s is that there seems to be a fair amount of people out there.

> Ward manager_London: Literally hundreds for every HCA post. So if they haven't been recruited that's probably because the ward sister has taken some decision not to, but no, it's not so difficult obviously we don't shortlist two hundred.

This plentiful supply of potential HCAs needs to be qualified in a number of respects. First, the local labour market conditions of the different Trusts had some impact on the flow of applicants. It has been noted that in Midlands, a relatively loose labour market provided the Trust with an opportunity to be more discriminating in their choices: this was manifest in the relatively high proportion of Midlands HCAs with previous health and social care experience.

Most interesting was South, where different labour market conditions were prevalent at the two Trust sites studied: in one, located in an area of high living costs and a fairly tight labour market, it remained quite difficult to recruit HCAs; in the other some 20 miles distant, both conditions were considerably relaxed ensuring an abundance of candidates. As a matron at the former site noted:

> Matron_South: We have real trouble recruiting healthcare assistants, good quality healthcare assistants ... at the moment our biggest vacancy factor is HCAs.

Second, some features of the HCA role were still perceived as unattractive, particularly in a tight labour market where potential applicants had options. Attention was drawn in particular to relative pay and its potential interaction with non-work pay benefits:

> Senior nurse_North: I think they're [HCAs] horrendously paid, I think the pay is absolutely awful.
> Ward manager_North: A lot of them are young people, single mums or single parents with kids and a lot of it's to do with benefits, you see, they've got to be really careful whether they're actually better off on benefits or working ... They're trying to figure out whether it's actually worth their while working, which most of the time it isn't. They're not paid enough, at a basic Band 2.

A fuller appreciation of labour supply can be gathered from exploring the backgrounds of those who actually became HCAs in our Trusts: in other words, who Trusts were successful in attracting to the role. The following background features are considered, in turn, in the following sections:

- personal characteristics;
- previous careers;
- motivations;
- engagement with the role reflected in patterns of work and employment.

Personal characteristics

HCAs share a number of personal characteristic which distinguish them from nurses, implying that across the health service a certain type of person is likely to take up the role. There are, however, differences in the personal make-up of the HCA workforce between Trusts, suggesting that local factors play some part in shaping the nature of this workforce. Table 5.4 sets out the personal background details of HCAs and registered nurses.

In terms of *shared characteristics*, in other words personal features found amongst HCAs in all four Trusts, the following points emerge:

- The overwhelming majority of HCAs are female, a feature they share with nurses.

- HCAs are distributed fairly evenly across the four age bands presented in Table 5.4, but they are relatively mature and significantly older than nurses. Around a third of HCAs are 50 years or more, but the proportion of nurses in this age range is much lower: in South and North, for example, the proportion of registered nurses above 50 is barely higher than 10 per cent. This difference in age profile is further reflected in the average age of the groups: the mean age of HCAs and nurses was respectively 42.6 and 38.4.

- HCAs are much less likely to have a black and minority ethnic (BME) background than nurses. In three of the four Trusts there is a statistically significant difference between HCAs and nurses in this respect. While around one half, and sometimes considerably more, of the nurse workforce in our Trusts had a BME background, the figure is invariably much lower for HCAs.

- A majority of HCAs, typically around three-quarters, have a partner and children. Nurses are as likely to have a partner but less likely to have children.

- A noteworthy minority of HCAs are the sole or main income earner, but nurses are more likely to assume primary earner status than HCAs.

- A considerable proportion of HCAs had attended a *local* primary school. Such attendance was seen as a proxy indicator for a strong connection to the local community. The proportion of HCAs attending a local primary school was a much higher than amongst nurses across all four Trusts, suggesting that HCAs are more firmly embedded in the area than their nurse colleagues.

A schematic presentation of the similarities between HCA and nurse personal characteristics is presented in Table 5.5 to provide a ready contrast been the two work groups.

Table 5.4 Personal background details of HCAs and nurses (%)

	South		Midlands		North		London		p-value	
	HCAs	Nurses	HCAs	Nurses	HCAs	Nurses	HCAs	Nurses	HCAs	Nurses
Age:										
Under 30 years	20	22	16	19	26	35	16	16	$\chi^2 = 6.82$, $p = 0.656$	$\chi^2 = 40.96$, $p < 0.001$
30s	23	47	25	29	21	28	24	37		
40s	26	19	26	35	27	24	27	23		
50 years or over	31	12	33	17	27	13	34	24		
Female	84	89	95	90	93	91	91	85	$\chi^2 = 13.27$, $p = 0.004$	$\chi^2 = 2.77$, $p = 0.428$
Ethnicity: BME	24	48	17	40	10	12	43	62	$\chi^2 = 40.56$, $p < 0.001$	$\chi^2 = 73.94$, $p < 0.001$
Married/living with long-term partner	75	78	83	80	78	68	80	83	$\chi^2 = 3.46$, $p = 0.326$	$\chi^2 = 8.94$, $p = 0.030$
Children	73	61	78	68	71	41	77	71	$\chi^2 = 2.50$, $p = 0.475$	$\chi^2 = 29.18$, $p < 0.001$
Sole or main income earner	31	43	46	49	31	49	44	44	$\chi^2 = 12.58$, $p = 0.006$	$\chi^2 = 1.88$, $p = 0.598$
Attended local primary school	42	18	69	58	54	39	34	22	$\chi^2 = 36.06$, $p < 0.001$	$\chi^2 = 71.53$, $p < 0.001$

Table 5.5 HCA–nurse background characteristics overview

	HCA	Nurse
Female	✓	✓
Young	✕	✓
BME	✕	✓
Partner	✓	✓
Children	✓	✕
Sole or main earner	✕	✓
Local primary school	✓	✕

While HCAs as a generic group differed from registered nurses in important respects, there were still some noteworthy *differences between HCAs* in the four Trusts:

- The proportion of HCAs with a BME background varied significantly between Trusts. In London, for example almost half had such a background, while in North the figure reached only 10 per cent. This pattern in part reflects the demographics of the two areas. London and North were Trusts located in areas with respectively the highest and lowest BME populations, and their different BME profiles might be seen as a further example of the HCA workforce reflecting the make-up of the local community (see Table 3.1).

- In South and North, HCAs were much less likely to be the sole or main income earner than those in Midlands and London: in the former Trust close to a third of HCAs fell into this category, while in the latter Trust it was over forty per cent.

- Trusts varied in terms of how deeply their HCA workforce was embedded in the local community. In Midlands, for instance, over two-thirds (69%) of HCAs had attended a local primary school, while in London the equivalent figure was barely over a third (34%). While HCAs were more connected to their local communities than nurses, clearly these HCA links to the locality still differed by trust

In short, HCAs in all four Trusts tended to be mature women, with partners and children, much less likely than nurses to have a BME background but considerably more likely to have a connection to the local community. At the same time, there remained some differences between HCAs in the respective Trusts. HCA workforces varied by ethnic diversity and connection to the community, suggesting the residual influence of local factors on the personal backgrounds of those attracted to the HCA role.

Career histories

In general, HCAs had diverse and often extensive career histories, suggesting that they brought to the role a breadth and depth of more or less relevant experience. These patterns were apparent in our HCA survey data, indicating important similarities in HCA career histories across our four cases, but again tempered by some variation between Trusts. Table 5.6 distinguishes sectors of potential HCA employment, and sets out the proportion of HCA with experience in them before taking up the HCA post. The bracketed figure represents the last sector of employment prior to assuming the HCA role.

The Table highlights the following similarities across Trusts:

- HCAs have previously been employed in a wide variety of sectors. Of those sectors listed, only finance and the utilities emerge as spheres where HCAs have had limited employment experience.

- Employment in the health and social care sectors are the most common areas of previous employment, with between a third and half of HCAs having worked there. A high proportion of HCAs also had work experience in retail, close to half in most Trusts, and to a lesser extent in manufacturing and leisure, typically around a quarter. Moreover, a noteworthy minority of

Table 5.6 Previous employment areas of HCAs (%)[a]

	South	**Midlands**	**North**	**London**
Healthcare	37 (19)	27 (14)	32 (20)	44 (29)
Social care	39 (24)	53 (47)	37 (28)	48 (33)
Education/child care	24 (11)	12 (4)	13 (9)	29 (9)
Voluntary or unpaid work	14 (1)	17 (1)	11 (1)	17 (0)
Retail	47 (13)	43 (15)	46 (15)	32 (10)
Manufacturing	26 (4)	41 (11)	26 (5)	21 (5)
Leisure	21 (8)	27 (4)	28 (8)	20 (5)
Finance	6 (3)	4 (1)	6 (3)	9 (1)
Utilities	3 (1)	1 (0)	2 (1)	0 (1)
Full-time carer at home	34 (5)	32 (2)	24 (5)	37 (4)
Other	19 (10)	6 (1)	9 (6)	8 (2)

[a] Figures in brackets provide the results for which area of work was the last before working as an HCA at their current Trust.

HCAs, typically a third or so, had been full-time unpaid carers in a domestic context.

- Despite this breadth of work experience, there were only a limited number of sectors providing a direct gateway into the HCA role. The most common sector of employment immediately prior to taking up the post (as indicated by the figures in brackets) is social care, closely followed by health. In all Trusts at least a fifth of HCAs had worked in either of these two sectors before taking up their HCA role. Few of the other sectors are an immediate port of entry into the HCA role. Although many HCAs have work experience in retail, manufacturing, and leisure, it is clear that they are seldom the last sector of employment before taking on the HCA role. Striking is the fact that few HCAs move directly from non-paid domestic care responsibilities to an HCA role: implicitly being a full-time mother is rarely a stepping stone to a job as an HCA.

There were some differences in career histories between Trusts:

- A relatively significant proportion of HCAs in London, close to half, had worked in both health and social care; almost two-thirds of HCAs worked in one of these sectors immediately prior to taking up the role, considerably higher than in South and North.

- Midlands draws on a comparatively high number of individuals with previous work experience in social care, typically employment in a care home. Around half worked in this sector immediately before taking up the HCA role, a finding which ties in with the earlier observation that loose local labour market conditions allowed Midlands to be fairly selective in its recruitment policy.

- HCAs at Midlands were also much more likely to have work experience in the manufacturing sector than those in other Trusts, a likely consequence of differences in the industrial structure of local economies.

Our qualitative data provided some confirmation of these findings but also gave further insights into the career trajectories of those who took up the HCA role. Drawing upon these qualitative data, it was possible to draft a map of the career journeys made by individual HCAs. The maps for the HCAs at two of our Trusts—South and Midlands—are set out below in Figures 5.1 and 5.2. These two trusts are drawn upon as examples of slightly different local labour markets: South having a somewhat tighter local labour market with higher living costs than Midlands. The maps use a slightly more refined set of sectors than covered in the survey. The thickness of arrows indicates the frequency with which a given path had been followed (the thicker the line the more HCAs had been down this path).

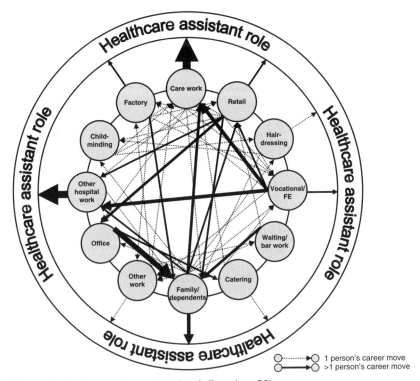

Figure 5.1 HCA career journeys at South Trust (n = 30).

Despite Trust differences in local labour market conditions, the two maps present very similar journeys for individuals into the HCA role, suggesting deep-rooted influences over the supply of HCAs which cut across the NHS. The maps reinforce the survey findings in highlighting limited gateways into the HCA role. They both confirm that employment in health and particularly social care remains the main entry points into the HCA role. At the same time while health and social care are the main entry points, breaking down the qualitative data in the two Trusts confirms that working outside of these sectors was commonly part of the career journeys.

Indeed, further refining these qualitative data allows a distinction to be made between three general paths in to the HCA role: a 'pure carer' path with previous employment solely in health or social care; a 'mixed' path where employment in these sectors has been combined with work in other non-caring sectors; and a 'non-care' path where the HCA had no work experience in health or social care. Table 5.7 reveals that in both Trusts the mixed path was by far the most common, over half moving along it into the HCA role.

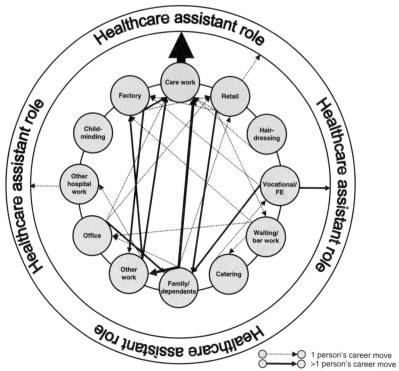

Figure 5.2 HCA career journeys at Midlands Trust (n = 16).

The two maps add to the survey data on career journeys in others ways: first, they vividly illustrate the considerable movement across diverse sectors of employment; second, they suggest some more common and established routes—some of the thicker lines include movement from office work to having and caring for children and then from non-paid caring for children to paid work; and finally, they highlight that once the HCA role is taken up it is not relinquished—neither of the maps has arrows back from HCA towards another sphere of employment (and back again to the HCA role).

Table 5.7 Career paths of HCAs

Career path	South (n = 30)	Midlands (n = 10)
Pure	7 (23%)	2 (20%)
Mixed	16 (53%)	6 (60%)
Non Care	7 (23%)	2 (20%)

The similarities between the two maps should not, however, detract from some noteworthy differences between them, confirming that career journeys display some sensitivity to local factors. Some career pathways are more firmly established in one Trust than the other. For example, it is striking that in South 'further education and vocational training' is a significant feeder into social care and health care work. In Midlands, however, education and training completely fail to connect to these sectors. Reinforcing the survey findings these maps also highlight the overwhelming importance of social care as an entry in to the HCA role in Midlands.

While the survey data and the maps provide a powerful insight into the patterns of career development amongst our HCAs, inevitably they are unable to capture the complete work and life journeys taken by individual HCAs which brought them to their current HCA role. The richness and diversity of these journeys can only fully be conveyed by full stories. Two such stories recounted by HCAs in interview are presented below. These stories are idiosyncratic or personal to the individual, but share certain features: the extended and convoluted character of the life and work journey; the movement between paid employment and often unpaid care work with family dependents; and the breadth and depth of experience implicitly brought to the HCA role:

> HCA_Midlands: I was fourteen when I left school. My first job, I worked as a waitress in a hotel with my mother, and then I went on to work in an office, then I got married, had a break, brought up five children, went back to work, about fifteen, about twenty years ago I went back to work. The first in a school, I worked in school kitchens … Then I went in to the care profession, I worked at a residential home looking after people with Alzheimer's disease. I was a senior carer there … and then I applied for a job here, I worked in orthopaedics, for eighteen months, and then in to the heart centre.
>
> HCA_London: I had a couple of little odd jobs and shops and that sort of thing, then I went in to work in a big factory where then obviously to have my two children when I didn't work while they were young, and I started working for the schools as in school dinner lady, playground duties, it fitted in with the school hours. Then I went from the school, I done a couple of, again a couple of the children were old enough, I went in to retail. Then I looked after my mum who'd had a stroke, and from then I decided I wanted to be in nursing, some role in nursing.

Motivation and aspirations

Motivation to take up a work role comprised a combination of 'push' factors, driving the individual out of their current job or situation, and 'pull' factors, encouraging movement towards a new post. However, while interaction between these two sets of factors might provide a stimulus for a shift in jobs, movement into a new work role was often underpinned by a deeper life narrative, a personal story, often informed by particular experiences and aspirations, which lent plausibility to the move. This section considers 'push' and 'pull' factors, and then life narratives.

Push factors

Across all Trusts there are examples of individuals becoming HCAs because they had been pushed out of their previous jobs. These push factors took various forms. There could be frustration with the routine nature of work in the previous role:

> HCA_South: I went to Sainsbury's because I thought I just wanted a job to earn a bit of extra money, that I could do it and go home. But I quickly found that I was extremely bored.

For others the work was not so much routine as 'depressing':

> HCA_Midlands: Working with the Alzheimer's. I mean for seven years I absolutely loved the job, and then it just got depressing because nobody ever got better and went home.

There were often concerns about the lack of opportunity and progression within the previous role:

> HCA_South: I was working in Burger King and supermarkets; it wasn't fulfilling in any way.
> HCA_Midlands: Working with the nursing home it was good but that was it, there was no future for me, anywhere to progress, so I applied to the Trust.

There could also be broader worries about the employing organization:

> HCA_Midlands: I just wasn't happy in doing what I was doing … I'd been in a residential home but moving in the nursing home was terrible … I just don't think they were very decent with the residents really.

Pull factors

The 'pull' factors might readily be seen as the 'other side of the coin' to the 'push' factors: the new job being regarded as a means of addressing concerns related to the former one. At the same time, individuals were drawn to the HCA role by what they viewed as its particular and distinctive attractions. There were some managerial concerns about these perceived attractions: a worry that potential applicants, drawing upon images and material from the media, might idealize or stereotype the role or inflate associated expectations, what some in the Trusts called the 'Holby City effect'.

Some HCAs felt the role was likely to be intrinsically rewarding: an opportunity to undertake fulfilling work:

> HCA_London: I wanted a bit more out of life, I wanted to make people better, to be honest.

HCA_Midlands: Working in a hospital is recognisable, it's hard work but at the end it's the prize you get from the patients when you do something, it's a rewarding job.

Partly related, others viewed a role in the NHS as being of worthy in its own right, a source of status, and perhaps security:

HCA_Midlands: I heard from somebody who worked here and she asked me what I'd feel about getting a job here and I said I'd love to work at the hospital: because it is quite hard to get a job like this around here.

The 'pull' of the HCA role also lay in its perceived convenience, not least in relation to the flexibility of its working hours—the possibility of part-time and shift working which aligned with domestic circumstances:

HCA_South: It was near home. It was easy to get to and I thought it would be nice to work in a hospital.

Life narratives

Most striking was the link between the motivation to become an HCA and more deeply rooted narratives, underpinning individual lives. These life narratives provided a plausible rationale and self-justification for taking up the HCA role, seeking to give effect to and signal certain aspirations. Three stories or narratives repeatedly emerged in our four Trusts founded on: 'reconnecting'; 'caring'; 'and nurse aspirations'.

A 'reconnecting' narrative This narrative was based on an individual's use of the HCA role to reconnect to a past nursing career. There were examples of former SENs who had returned to secondary healthcare in an HCA capacity. More common were HCAs with an overseas background who had trained and often qualified as nurses in their country of origin, and were using the HCA role to 'mark time' as they sought to gain registered status in the UK:

HCA_Midlands: In the Philippines I was a registered nurse and then I worked in a hospital in the medical surgical ward there. I came here 2003, so at least nine years I was working in the hospital, and then after that, because my husband was hired by this hospital back home because his specialties are more on cardio as well. So ... he got me and my family so I work here. And then before I work here I was working in one of the nursing homes in [local town] ... for almost two years as well.

A 'caring narrative' A considerable number of HCAs had a recent care experience or episode, typically in their personal lives, which informed their decision to become an HCA. Looking after an elderly or sick relative or a friend had provided a stimulus to seek more formal and regular employment in care work. For some the provision of care in a domestic context also sparked an appreciation of personal capability. For others such a care episode prompted a recognition that care work could be intrinsically rewarding:

> HCA_South: My husband became ill in 1991 and I looked after him, he had terminal cancer. After he died I went back in to a salon for a couple of years work, but it had changed so much since I started salon work that I didn't like it anymore. And there was an advertisement in a local paper advertising an open day to a care home and Mum said to me why don't you go because I'd looked after my husband.
>
> HCA_London: I was unemployed for about three months between there and here and in that three months my uncle was dying of prostrate cancer. He was living in a one bedroom flat that was in a high-rise and I wasn't having none of it because nobody was going in to him until three or four o'clock in the afternoon. So I got in my car … I put him in my car and brought him home, and he died with me at home. And that kind of flipped me to want to come and do this, and that was the start of my medical career.
>
> HCA_London: They actually said it was a urine infection for six weeks, and when they bothered to take a blood test [from my husband] they realised how seriously ill he was. So my life kind of got put on hold for the following, probably near enough two years he was in and out, well mostly in hospital. They started the chemo treatment … They basically turned it around and they managed to save him … I'd seen a different side of it having him being so poorly and spending so long at the hospital, it's what I wanted to do.

An 'aspirational nurse' narrative

Many HCAs had taken on the role as a proxy for a career in registered nursing or as a stepping stone towards it. This was often rooted in a longstanding but unfulfilled desire to become a nurse:

> HCA_South: I always wanted to become a nurse but having very little confidence in myself, by the time I was twelve I'd convinced myself I was not going to be good enough for a nursing job and decided to go for something else. And then I grew up, I got my qualifications and so it sort of occurred to me, hang on a second I can do this.
>
> HCA_North: When I left school I went to college and I did a BTEC diploma in caring, because I did intend to go into nursing, but at the time my mum was, my mum got sick. So I had to look after her for awhile and it all got put on the, the backburner basically, it all got shelved. And then I ended up working in a casino as a croupier.
>
> London_HCA: Ever since I was going to school I wanted to be a nurse, and that was my idea of being a nurse. But because of my mum dying at a young age, when I was sixteen years of age, and she was only thirty-six when I lost my mum. So at the time I was starting to do shorthand and typing. When I come to this country I wanted to do nursing.

The prevalence and potency of this aspirational nurse narrative as a rationale for becoming an HCA is further reflected in the survey findings. These reveal that in all the Trusts around half of HCAs had nurse aspirations prior to taking up the role (see Table 5.8).

Table 5.8 Nursing ambition *prior* to HCA role (%)

	South	Midlands	North	London	p-value
Nursing ambition	43	43	47	59	$\chi^2 = 6.82$, $p = 0.078$

Work and employment pattern

The final dimension of HCA backgrounds relates to patterns of employment—their length of service at the Trusts, their distribution between pay bands, their formal qualifications, and their patterns of work-hours and shifts.

These background details on the work and employment conditions of HCAs reveal some important similarities between Trusts, again tempered by some equally noteworthy differences. Table 5.9 sets out the working patterns of HCAs and once more compares them with nurses as a means of establishing whether or not they are distinctive.

Table 5.9 reveals that in terms of length of service, HCAs are fairly experienced: the average length of HCA service is nine years and only around a quarter of HCAs in any given Trust have less than two years service. In most of the Trusts around a third of HCAs have ten or more years' service. In these respects, HCAs are not too dissimilar to the nurses, whose average length of service was also nine years. This is slightly at odds with some of the qualitative findings, which suggest that HCAs are perceived as the mainstay of wards, less likely to move than nurses, and consequently more likely to be a source of ward-based knowledge and continuity:

> Manager_London: When I was a student nurse, the healthcare assistants were the ones that absolutely knew what was going on, were incredible, usually stayed in one place for a long time, much longer than any qualified nurses so knew the running of the ward, knew what was expected, had that intuition, if you like, of, 'Oh, you know, that patient's not quite right', sort of that, that sort of expert in people skills....On the whole they do tend to stay in one place for a long time, it's massively important.

HCAs were more readily distinguishable from nurses in terms of flexible working, particularly part-time working. Part-time working amongst HCAs was not especially prevalent, only around a quarter in each Trust worked fewer than 29 hours a week. In all Trusts, however, HCAs are significantly more likely to work part-time than nurses, a finding which might be related to the greater childcare responsibilities of HCAs (see earlier section):

> HCA_London: I joined here permanent bank full time, then I was requested by one of my ward managers a long time ago to join the staff, and I said I couldn't do it because I needed to accommodate with the children's hours and family-friendly. She agreed, and it carried on until this day and they were accommodating on the ward, I'll be very

Table 5.9 Work background details of HCAs and nurses (%)

	South		Midlands		North		London		p-value	
	HCAs	Nurses	HCAs	Nurses	HCAs	Nurses	HCAs	Nurses	HCAs	Nurses
Length of service:										
Less than 2 years	29	24	25	14	26	19	27	25		
2–4 years	27	21	13	14	13	23	14	13	$\chi^2 = 21.43$, $p = 0.044$	$\chi^2 = 33.42$, $p = 0.001$
5–9 years	21	36	29	37	24	21	29	33		
10–19 years	14	12	19	15	22	15	19	14		
20 years or more	10	8	15	20	15	22	11	15		
Part-time (up to 29 hours)	29	16	26	15	25	11	14	10	$\chi^2 = 8.26$, $p = 0.041$	$\chi^2 = 3.30$, $p = 0.348$
Shifts worked in last month:										
Early	82	80	77	66	61	67	84	82	$\chi^2 = 25.22$, $p < 0.001$	$\chi^2 = 16.84$, $p = 0.001$
Late	67	78	66	60	56	61	77	80	$\chi^2 = 13.09$, $p = 0.004$	$\chi^2 = 26.14$, $p < 0.001$
Night	44	65	63	63	68	64	68	69	$\chi^2 = 25.20$, $p < 0.001$	$\chi^2 = 0.99$, $p = 0.802$
All three shift types worked in last month	30	51	42	38	41	42	56	58	$\chi^2 = 19.36$, $p < 0.001$	$\chi^2 = 13.50$, $p = 0.004$

honest with you, I tend to request my off-duty and there's give and take and I'm happy.

Patterns of shift working were more idiosyncratic to Trusts. In three Trusts (South, Midlands, and North) working all three shifts is a minority practice amongst HCAs, a pattern they shared with nurses. Again this relates to HCAs (and perhaps nurses) working shifts which fit in with their domestic circumstances:

> HCA_South: I didn't want to be an HCA, [but] the driving impetus was that it fitted around my family hours; that it was available … It wasn't a role I looked for and it never has been. I was comfortable and I could earn a living and its something I'm okay at doing.

There was, however, some variation between the Trusts as to whether HCAs were more or less likely to work all three shifts than nurses. In terms of the shift patterns worked London stood out. It can be seen that in this trust the majority of HCAs, and indeed nurses, worked all three shifts. This finding relates to the recent introduction of an e-rostering system in this Trust and points to the efficacy of a local practice designed to standardize and regularize shift working across the ward team.

Summary

The general pattern to emerge from this review of HCA backgrounds across the dimensions highlighted—personal characteristics, work and life experience, motivation and aspirations, employment and working arrangements—is one of differences and similarities between Trusts. The demand for and supply of HCAs has been seen as sensitive to local Trust factors. Local catchment areas do vary in terms of their labour markets, and their industrial and demographic make-up, in ways which impact on those taking up the HCA role. Moreover, differences in Trust policies and practices also emerge as shaping the level and nature of the HCA intake. However, more striking are the significant commonalities in HCA backgrounds across the four Trusts, suggesting the influence of cross-cutting, deep-seated, and powerful structural features associated with the HCA role and the NHS workforce.

In terms of personal characteristics, HCAs were revealed as distinctive from the nurses they work alongside in a number of important respects. While both groups were mainly made up of women with partners, HCAs were more likely to be rooted in the local community, to be older, and to have children, while being less likely to be the sole or main household earner and have a BME background. The distinctiveness of HCAs in these terms raises the possibility that this group of workers does bring novel experiences, skills, and capabilities to the care process.

This possibility is heightened by the breadth of life and work experiences HCAs bring to the role. The quantitative and qualitative data highlighted similarities in the operation of local labour markets for HCAs in the Trusts, noteworthy in the absence of workforce regulation associated with this occupation. Those drawn to the HCA role had diverse employment backgrounds, with previous periods of work in a range of different sectors. However, a limited number of career paths for these workers were also uncovered, with Trusts implicitly establishing select gateways into the HCA role: thus, typically employment in health and social was the most direct route into work as an HCA.

HCAs were presented as driven towards the role by a range of push factors, largely associated with the frustrations of previous work. They were attracted by various pull factors, encouraging a belief in the fulfilling or convenient nature of the HCA role. However, individuals were often motivated to become an HCA as part of a life narrative, a personal story which lent plausibility to the decision to take on the role. Three such narratives consistently emerged, connecting the role to: previous experience of the nurse profession; episodes of unpaid care work; and long-standing nurse aspirations. The life narrative associated with nurse aspirations, in particular, relates to a view of the HCA role as a stepping stone into registered nursing. It is a narrative which chimes with a public policy interest in using the HCA role to increase workforce, particularly registered nurse, capacity in the NHS.

There were signs that working arrangements across all four Trusts had been crafted to the needs of individual HCAs. Shift patterns and hours of working displayed some irregularity and a lack of standardization, suggesting that individuals moulded the role to their needs and circumstances: a not insignificant minority of HCAs worked on a part-time basis, certainly a higher proportion than nurses, while, with the exception of one Trust, only a minority of HCAs worked all three shift, implying some 'cherry picking'. At the same time it might be argued that these flexible working arrangements were a trade-off against the low pay received by HCAs: in all of our Trusts the HCA workforce was overwhelmingly a Band 2 workforce. In short, HCAs were concentrated in the lowest of the HCA bands. This pattern of employment raises some interesting issues on the relationship between pay, qualifications, and, by implication, capabilities. These are issues which we consider in further detail in Chapter 7 dealing with the impact of the HCA role on post holders.

Issues for reflection

The findings in this chapter suggest the need for Trusts to consider:

- Introducing tighter entry requirements and recruit higher-quality individuals to HCA posts where labour markets in the Trust's catchment area are loose, and the supply of potential HCA candidate is high.

- Emphasizing the intrinsic rewards of the HCA role, in particular the scope to 'make a difference', as a means of attracting strong candidates to the role.

- The limited gateways into the role: if Trusts are seeking individuals with more diverse work experience, they should seek to broaden their recruitment efforts; if they are content with entry through these gateways they should adopt more targeted approaches to recruitment.

- The aspirations of those selected for the HCA role as a means of more efficiently and effectively managing their career development.

- The different life narratives of those drawn to become HCAs as a way of assessing how they might engage with the role.

- Practices for delivering NVQ qualifications: where Trusts devote energy, focus, and resources to NVQs, there are marked differences in the proportion of HCAs with NVQ qualifications.

- The consequences of narrowly concentrating HCAs within pay Band 2.

Chapter 6

The shape and nature of the healthcare assistant role

HCA_South: I might be called a healthcare assistant but really, truly I do it all on my own. So I don't really assist, they [nurses] assist me in a way because it's my job to clean and freshen up patients.

Introduction

A job title typically provides few clues to the nature and variety of tasks in practice performed by the post holder. One field of study, industrial relations, has been predicated on the view that the employment relationship is incomplete (Marsden, 1999; Martin, 2003). The formal means for describing and prescribing the occupational requirements to be delivered by the employee in return for a given reward are difficult, if not impossible, to codify through any formal means such as a contract of employment or a job description. These formal mechanisms can never meaningfully tie down or stipulate the myriad situations or work needs associated with the enactment of a work role. In short, an occupation-in-action defies ready or straightforward definition as to its shape, contour, and content. Such a perspective raises questions about the process by which tasks and responsibilities are allocated to an occupational role—the factors influencing this process and their interaction—and the forms assumed by the role—a single job title being unlikely to capture variation in the configuration of activities emerging in response to shifting needs and circumstances.

It follows that a reliance on the 'healthcare assistant' job title is likely to provide only a flawed and partial view of the substantive form assumed by this role. Indeed, it might be argued that in the case of the HCA the link between job title, tasks, and responsibilities is particularly opaque. We have seen that the role has evolved over many years, and has been subject to a variety of public policy iterations on the delivery of health and nursing care. In this context, the various labels attached to the nurse support role are more likely to be the source of uncertainty rather than clarity as to tasks performed. Certainly there is a sequencing of job titles—nurse auxiliary, healthcare assistant, and clinical support workers—tied to public policy developments, and possibly suggesting some differences in the nature of the role. But the contemporary use of these varied terms makes it difficult to discern whether they denote a difference in substance, or simply a different label for the same role.

This chapter seeks to explore the shape and nature of the role in practice. This will be pursued in three ways:

1. *Searching for the core of role*. Whilst noting the scope for variation in the form assumed by the HCA role, it remains open to consideration whether the role has a core: in others words, whether it has an irreducible essence, with post holders sharing certain key attributes or performing a set of shared tasks. This issue was considered through broad perceptions of the role: who the HCA was actually supporting and what makes a 'good' HCA.

2. *Contingent influences on the shape of the role*. An acknowledgement that the HCA role might assume different forms encourages a search for the range of contingent factors influencing its shape and contours, particularly as it extends beyond the core. This issue was investigated in a grounded way, using the qualitative material to uncover these influential factors and the means by which they affected the nature of the HCA role. In examining these factors a broad distinction is made between influences related to structure and to agency.

   Structural influences are founded on the view that there may be powerful systems, rules, and practices, which determine the shape of the HCA role. These structural influences might be found at different levels and be driven by various considerations. In part they have been built into the design of this research: thus it has been suggested that shared Trust approaches to the shape of the HCA role across the four Trusts might well point to forces underpinning workforce structure in the NHS which lead to convergence. Moreover, differences in the contours of the HCA role between clinical areas similarly might indicate the determining influence, say, of patient conditions on the tasks required from post holders.

   The influence of agency draws attention to the discretion and choice available to stakeholders in shaping the HCA role. Agency might well be complementary to structure in the sense that structure constrains but does not necessarily determine. Again agency might be found at different levels. While some doubts were raised about the strategic orientation of Trusts towards the HCA role, difference in the choice and application of policies might be seen to influence the shape of the role. At a micro level, attention has already been drawn to the crafting of working patterns by individual HCA post holders; equally such crafting might extend to the tasks performed by HCAs, linked perhaps to their personal aspirations and orientations to the role.

3. *Types of HCA: mapping contours and unpacking substance*. Building on this grounded picture of contingent influences, consideration needs to be given to the substantive form assumed by the role, the range of tasks performed by post holders, and the different ways in which these might be configured. In the main, a quantitative approach was used to explore these issues. A survey was designed to develop a more organized and systematic view of the different types of HCA role, based on the configuration of tasks performed. These same survey data were also used to further consider the influence of structure and agency: whether different types of HCAs might be associated with the respective factors.

The chapter is divided in to three main parts, reflecting these areas of interest. They reflect the sequence of data collection, and therefore highlight the development of our analytical approach. Drawing upon qualitative data, the first presents findings on the core of the HCA role: who the HCA supports and what makes a 'good' HCA. Also relying on qualitative data, the second sets out the range of influences shaping the HCA role. The qualitative findings fed into our nurse and HCA questionnaire design, and the third part uses the survey data to explore different types of HCA role. The chapter highlights the varied forms assumed by the HCA role and suggests that structure and agency combine to influence the types of HCA to be found within and between Trusts.

Searching for the core

The locus of support

Interviewees were asked a broad, open question asking them to outline the role of the HCA. Responses to this question varied both in terms of the approach taken to answering the question as well as in relation to its substance. Some respondents immediately homed-in on the specific tasks performed by the HCA. Others chose to focus on their personal experiences: 'I'd say it was hard work'; or responded normatively: 'We're the hardest workers' or 'general dogsbody really'. Some found it difficult to tie down the role, often seeing it as contingent: 'it depends on the individual'. Nonetheless, the role was often defined in terms of precisely who the HCA was supporting: the nurse, the patient, or, in a more general sense, the team. These were not mutually exclusive options, in acting as nurse support or patient support the HCA is, after all, acting as a team support as well:

> Senior nurse_Midlands: [The role is] to support the trained nurse, to be there for the patient as well as the trained nurses. I always believe that you work as a team.
> Ward manager_London: The main role I think is to be part of the team, to work alongside the nurse, to work with the patient to be seen to be working with the patients. I don't see the role of the healthcare assistant as somebody who's just doing all the washes, taking the commodes, that's not what they're there for, they're there to be counted, to be seen and to be valued and not to be given all the menial jobs.

Indeed, it was a fairly common response to link support for the nurse with support for the patient:

> Matron_London: The role of the HCA, is somebody to help with the patients' basic care, to perform observations: temperature, blood pressure, pulse and respirations. To assist the trained nurse in duties, for example, they may assist in dressings but not actually do the dressings themselves.

However, typically respondents presented a primary locus of HCA support, stressing that HCAs were essentially assisting the nurse or the patient or the team. These different emphases might be viewed as giving some sense of where the role's core lay.

There were some patterns in the perceived locus of support from different actors. Nurses were somewhat more likely to regard the HCA as supporting them, whereas the ward manager viewed the HCA as supporting the team, and the HCAs saw themselves as supporting the patient. These patterns were not, however, hard-and-fast and are worth dwelling on in a little more detail.

Most commonly the HCA was presented as a *support for the nurse*, with considerable emphasis placed on the HCA as relieving the nurse of certain elements of direct care provision:

> Matron_Midlands: They're [HCAs] fundamentally supporting the trained nurse; in terms of direction and instruction that is from the trained nurse, so it's supportive.
> Ward manager_North: [The HCA role is] to support the qualified nurse. To me it'll be to concentrate on the fundamentals of care which are the basic: your hygiene needs and anything that your patient needs, making sure they're fed, making sure they're sat up for breakfast, helping with the bed areas and general cleanliness of the ward. And taking it on from there, being aware of pressure areas and working with the qualified nurses.
> Nurse_London: It's to support the trained nurse in carrying out the duties, but we can't do everything, so we need somebody to be able to help out and do it, and do the bits we can't do.

Although less common, some interviewees placed greater emphasis on the HCA *as a support for the patient*:

> HCA_South: Because of the title, whether we're a healthcare assistant or clinical support worker, I feel that I need to come in and care for the patient's needs, help them if they need to feed, help them with their washing and dressing and their mobilisation as well.
>
> HCA_North: My job involves looking after patients with the help of a qualified nurse and look after the ward with the help of qualified nurse, because I am joined with qualified nurse here, that's my role, look after patients.

A few respondents placed the primary emphasis on the HCA as a team resource, a somewhat different perspective to the nurse and patient support perspectives in perhaps understating any claim of ownership of the role by any given stakeholder:

> Ward manager_London: They're a fairly valuable member of our team actually are healthcare assistants, because … patients being quite dependent but also can be very sick as well, you know, they're very, oh how can I put them into words really?
>
> HCA_South: It's to care for the patients and to support the other members of the team, so that everyone works as a team together.
>
> Ward manager_North: They're an important part of the team. They might not think they are sometimes but I think they're the ones that are going to stay long-term and in a way we should be maybe investing more in to them.

The 'good' HCA

In considering the nature of the HCA role, stakeholders—HCAs, nurses, and ward managers—were asked an open interview question about the qualities they felt a 'good' HCA needed. This question was also raised in the patient focus groups. It is a question which seeks to address the essence of the HCA role: the attributes of the 'good' HCA are likely to reflect its core purpose. Table 6.1 reveals the findings to this question: the responses have been presented under a limited number of attributes which, in a generic sense, capture the wide range of often overlapping qualities voiced by interviewees.

In comparison with the findings on the locus of support, the table suggests a slightly different emphasis on where the essence of the HCA role lies. The need for the 'good' HCA to be 'caring' and 'compassionate' appears to place the patient at the centre of the HCAs' concerns: well over half the HCAs and over a third of the nurses and ward managers viewed these attributes as essential to the 'good HCA', with patients also seeing these capabilities as central. At the same time, there are some noteworthy differences of emphasis between these different stakeholders. Perhaps reflecting the weight placed by HCAs on supporting the patient, 'caring' and 'compassion' are by far the most common feature cited by HCAs as characterizing the 'good' HCA'. Whilst nurses also

Table 6.1 The 'good' HCA (%)

	HCA (n = 72)	Nurse (n = 49)	Ward manager (n = 27)	Total (n = 148)	Patient focus groups
Caring/compassion	58	35	37	47	✓
Communication	26	31	30	28	
Team orientated/flexible	24	20	44	26	
Enjoys/motivation/committed	24	18	44	26	
Friendly/approachable/listens	21	18	33	22	✓
Patience/tolerance/empathy	26	16	4	19	✓
Knows limits/follows instructions	10	20	22	16	✓
Initiative	8	22	11	14	
Sense of humour	14	8	19	13	✓

frequently mention these features as marking the 'good HCA', 'communication' and 'initiative' are not too far behind, attributes the nurse might hope and expect to find amongst HCAs principally oriented to support them. Ward managers have an even more distinctive set of 'desired' HCA attributes, again alluding to a distinctive view of the HCA: in line with an interest in the HCA as a team member, close to half of the ward managers include a 'team orientation' in their list of HCA attributes.

An extended role

Despite some difference of emphasis between stakeholders, a considerable degree of consensus across the Trusts emerged to suggest that the core of the HCA role lay in indirect and direct patient care: in other words the essence of the role was seen as bedside and patient centred:

> Ward manager_London: They provide basic nursing care. They're there to help wash people, they are there to do jobs in an emergency. I don't think it's necessarily always part of their job to do observations, that's one of the jobs I think that they get palmed off with.

Equally, there were suggestions that the provision of direct care—washing and feeding—marked a shift in the core, with the more traditional nursing auxiliary previously confined to indirect tasks such as bed making and other ancillary tasks. As one manager who had once been an HCA notes:

> Manager_London: When I first started doing HCA work you were never there for a handover because that was the trained nurse's job, so you could go and deal with a patient that you knew absolutely nothing about. Whereas these days you're more involved with the care and I actually think that they've started to notice that HCAs do more of the care for the patient than sometimes a lot of the staff nurses do.

At the same time, it was apparent that across the Trusts, the HCA role was moving to take on more extended tasks. Certainly the limits of the HCA role were clearly drawn in all Trusts: for example, the dispensation of any medication remained the sole prerogative of the registered nurse, but before this limit was reached, a range of more complex and technical tasks such as taking observations, performing ECGs and taking bloods could be performed by HCAs:

> Ward manager_North: [HCAs] do the observations on here. They're not solely responsible for the observations but I think the reality is that they do the observations more than the qualified nurses do now because of the turnover of patients and the paperwork and everything else that the qualified nurses do.
>
> Manager_London: As qualified practitioners' roles have changed with regards to taking on new skills, the same has happened for healthcare assistants. So a lot more has been expected of them [HCAs] with regards to things they now undertake, so it might be that they've been trained up to do venapuncture.

This presentation of the HCA role as essentially revolving around direct as well as indirect patient care, but with signs of extension beyond these core areas, suggests that a broad space is opening up for its performance: a space within which there is a considerable overlap between the tasks undertaken by HCAs and nurses. In practice, the division of nursing labour within this space remains very much an empirical question. Our observation of HCAs and nurses at work provided a means of exploring this issue: it allowed an assessment of how similar or different the respective roles were in relation to these various types of task. Figure 6.1 draws upon our observational data to compare the relative proportion of the shift spent by HCAs and nurses on different types of activity. Definitions and examples of the five task categories are provided in Chapter 3.

The figure provides strong confirmation that HCAs rather than registered nurses provide much of the direct and indirect care to patients. HCAs were spending a considerable proportion of their time on these areas, around 60 per cent of the shift. While nurses had not completely deserted this ground, spending close to a third of their shift on it, they were much less engaged in such care than HCAs. The suggestion that HCAs had significantly extended their role beyond this patient-centred direct care work finds less support from

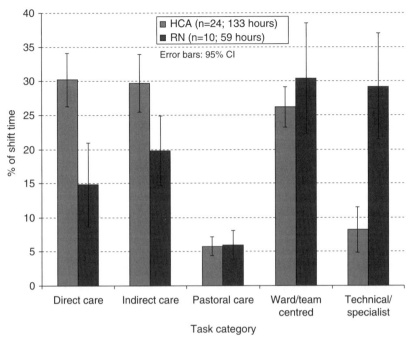

Figure 6.1 Observed shape of the HCA role: HCAs versus nurses (early shift only).

these findings. The time spent by HCAs on direct patient care was taken up by registered nurses in performing technical and specialist tasks not typically performed by HCAs: while nurses spent close to a third of their shift on such tasks, HCAs devoted considerable less than ten per cent of their time to them. Ward- and team-centred tasks, as well as pastoral care, appeared to be largely shared between the two groups.

There remains a need to 'drill-down' into this general picture. For example, there were suggestions that the nature of the HCA role was subject to considerable variation. As a ward manager from North noted:

> Ward manager_North: [The HCA role is] different wherever you are and dependent on the skill set of the individual. It's also down to how the individual's motivated and in terms of what they want to take on. Sometimes it's being clear what is the role, and that's different everywhere you go in relation to if you talk to somebody about a health assistant in one place, a nurse assistant somewhere else, they're different. It's fine them being different if they're different for a reason, but you can be different in one medical ward to another, it can be the whim of the ward sister, those types of things. .

This quote highlights the range of structural and personal influences shaping the HCA role. The next section considers these influences in a more systematic way.

Contingent influences on the shape of the HCA role

The tasks and responsibilities of the HCA were typically set out in a job description. These were, however, invariably drafted in broad terms: in Midlands, for example the Band 2 job description comprised over 20 separate tasks. In practice, the take up and configuration of these and other tasks were determined by the interaction of a variety of workplace, structural, and behavioural factors. This produced considerable variation in the contours and substance of the HCA role. As a manager in London noted:

> Manager_London: Although there's some generic job descriptions, the senior sisters on the ward are, rightly or wrongly, left to use their staff in the way that they want to. So you'll find across the Trust different HCA groups are doing different things and working in different ways. So some are more autonomous than others and have a wider skill set than others.

The qualitative research highlighted four sets of factors with a significant influence on the configuration of tasks performed by the HCA. These factors are set out in Figure 6.2. Those related to the Trust, the ward, and the clinical setting might be seen as being predominantly structural; those associated with the individual imply a degree of personal agency. Each set of influences is considered in turn.

Trust

Any given Trust has at its disposal a range of policies and practices which might be used to shape the HCA role. Substantive and procedural variation in

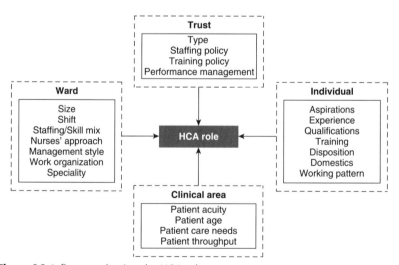

Figure 6.2 Influences shaping the HCA role.

the use of these levers between hospitals might account for differences in the nature of the role. Most obviously, there is scope to develop job descriptions which set parameters to the role, but in a stronger sense, pay systems, training, and performance management arrangements might be used to influence the willingness and ability of HCAs to undertake certain tasks.

In contrast to many parts of the economy, the NHS has national systems, mainly articulated through Agenda for Change (AfC) and the Knowledge and Skills Framework (KSF), standardizing the form assumed by these levers. This did not, however, detract from the possibility of Trusts using these levers to manage workforces in a distinctive way in pursuit of specific Trust goals; indeed AfC and the KSF were viewed by national policymakers as being designed for such a purpose. However, at the level of the Trust, these systems emerged as providing only a 'light touch' influence on the shape of the HCA role. This has already been highlighted in the discussion of strategic approaches to the HCA role. However, it is worth restating that across the four Trusts, the limited use of such human resource levers to shape the HCA role in the context of broader hospital aims ensured a highly permissive corporate regime. The effect was to allow other, lower-level, forces to hold sway in the shaping the HCA role, sometimes in idiosyncratic, occasionally in disordered ways.

Beyond the clear rules on the dispensation of medication, corporate systems to regulate what HCAs could and could not do were not greatly in evidence. In two Trusts—London and South—policy documents had been published on the management of the HCA role. At South this document took the form of a Code of Practice, produced for HCAs in 2002, and, in London, guidance on the principles of delegation to HCAs had been published in 2003. These documents set out broad principles designed to regulate the shape and management of the HCA role. In London, for example, the guidance noted that:

> The HCA will at all times:
> - recognise any limitations of competence and only carry out those tasks which are included in the job description for which formal training and assessment have been undertaken;
> - be aware that they should make the practitioner aware if the task is beyond their competence;
> - have responsibility for care delivery.

However, there was limited awareness of these principles amongst interviewees in these Trusts, and few if any attempts to monitor or enforce their application.

This corporate permissiveness was most in evidence in reviewing the relationship between the pay band, the NVQ qualification, and the tasks performed by HCAs. In all four Trusts this relationship had broken down.

For example, in exploring the relationship between banding and NVQ level, a manager in London stated:

> Manager_London: It's all over the place. It's historical and, again, I think it's because there's that many different departments, that many different wards, they all have their own job descriptions. Again it's, 'Oh you've been here so many years you need a Band 3', you know.

The misalignment between pay, qualification, and role is considered in much more detail in Chapter 7, exploring the management of HCAs. But on the evidence presented, it would be fair to suggest that Trust policies and practices only played a limited part in shaping the HCA role in a clear and organized way.

Clinical area

Differences between clinical areas—general surgical and general medical—in terms of the patients admitted and their conditions were seen to affect the nature of the HCA role. A surgical ward will require considerable movement of patients to and from the theatre, while a national 18-week limit on waiting time filtered down to place pressure on patient discharge. In some surgical wards with High Dependency Unit (HDU) step-down beds, patients were naturally in need of quite acute and specialist care, requiring a richer skill/grade mix. Medical wards, particularly those taking elderly patients, were likely to have a slightly higher age profile with more confused patients, often with chronic conditions, needing considerable ongoing care and support.

The analysis of the observation data provides some support for the view that the clinical area influences the nature of the HCA role. As can be seen from Figure 6.3, HCAs in medical wards were spending more of their shift on the provision of direct care than those in surgical wards—respectively around a third compared to a quarter of their time—while devoting more of their time to indirect and technical/specialist tasks.

More striking were differences in the pattern and rhythm of the HCA role across the shift in different clinical areas. Figures 6.4 and 6.5 present the flow of tasks across the early morning shifts respectively, in the surgical and medical wards at our four Trusts. Each series of points plotted on these figures indicates the proportion of time spent on the different activities by HCAs during their shift. The patterns present different rhythms of activity in the two clinical areas: after a similar handover period, a team activity, attended by HCAs, on the medical ward direct care is quickly established and sustained as the key HCA activity for much of the shift until near lunchtime when blood monitoring is undertaken. By contrast, on the surgical ward, a burst of direct care at the beginning of the shift, associated with getting patients out of bed and washing

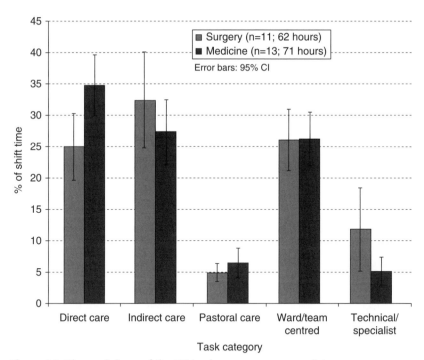

Figure 6.3 Observed shape of the HCA role: surgery versus medicine (early shift only).

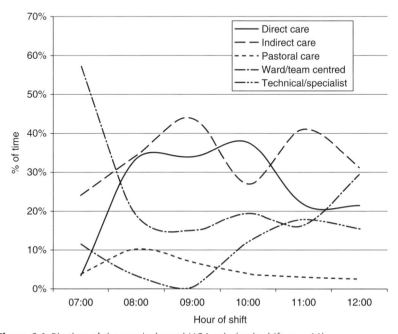

Figure 6.4 Rhythm of the surgical ward HCA role (early shift, n = 11).

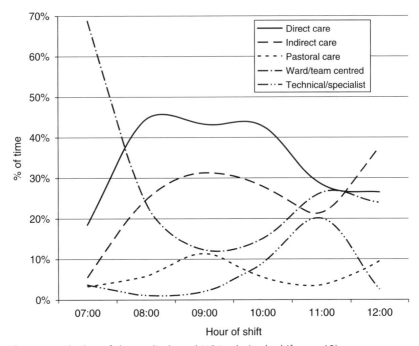

Figure 6.5 Rhythm of the medical ward HCA role (early shift, n = 13).

them, gives way to an ebb and flow of different types of indirect and team-related tasks.

This relationship between clinical areas, the nature and condition of a patient and the role of an HCA is further explained by a matron at North, who notes that differences in the discharge process lead HCAs to play a much greater role in the delivery of direct patient care in medical wards, in this case covering the elderly, than in surgical wards:

> Matron_North: Doing discharges from an elderly ward is a really complex thing that takes up a lot of a qualified nurse's time, so I think it's important you've got the role of the healthcare there to provide the basic nursing care. Across in surgery, you know, the discharge of a patient is picking up a phone, there's nothing complex there. So I think we could utilise the role of the healthcare in a more proficient way like the doctors' assistants, you know, for the phlebotomy, for the venflons.

Ward

The shape of the HCA role was heavily influenced by a number of features associated with the organization and management of the ward. These features included the shift, work organization, ward workforce, and management style.

Shift

The structure and nature of a ward shift had a powerful effect on the shape of the HCA role. Tasks and responsibilities undertaken were highly sensitive to whether the shift was in the morning, afternoon, or night. In the main, the respective shifts had a standardizing effect, generating their own routines, requirements, and interactions across all wards and areas regardless of speciality.

The early shift was generally perceived as the most intense: HCAs were required to help patients out of bed as well as wash them and cope with two meals times, breakfast and lunch. In contrast, the late shift overlapped with visiting times and ensured a much greater interaction with the patients' friends and relatives. The night shift was often the quietest of the shifts, but could be unpredictably intense: staffing levels were at their lowest, so that if problems did arise they could generate considerable pressure. These differences in shift activity meant that an HCA working only nights, for example, would be performing a role shaped very differently to an HCA, say, working just day shifts.

Work organization

There was some variation in the organization of work on the ward, which could impact on the nature of the HCA role. In general, there were three models of work organization on wards: a fairly fixed model based on a team covering a given number of bays, the HCA working with the nurses as part of this team; a more flexible model, the HCA working in a more fluid fashion across the whole of the ward and with nurses as and when needed; and a bay-centred model, the HCA having responsibility for a single, given bay. These different models shaped the HCA role in different ways, for example, the team model would see the HCA working with a more limited and fixed set of patients and nurses than a flexible model; with responsibility for a given bay, the HCA would have a focused set of ongoing, monitoring tasks.

Ward workforce

At various times during any given shift, a range of occupational groups will be working on the ward alongside the HCA. The list of such occupations is extensive, including housekeepers, ward assistants, cleaners, caterers, porters, student nurses, physiotherapists, phlebotomists, physicians' assistants, and occupational therapists. To varying degrees, the activities of these groups overlapped with those performed by the HCAs: for example, the student will engage in aspects of direct and indirect care and the physiotherapist might ask the HCA to help walk a patient

The presence or not of such groups on the ward had an impact on the tasks performed by the HCA: regular visits by a phlebotomist clearly reduced opportunities for HCAs to take blood. As highlighted in our observation the presence of a ward assistant also affected the shape of the HCA role:

> Field note_Midlands (Medical): It was noticeable how much more time the [HCAs] had because of the WA [ward assistant] doing the drinks round and breakfast. It meant they could rattle through their washes without interruption. The observee did remark that Wednesdays was her least favourite shift because the WA didn't work that day and as a consequence it was a lot busier.

The use of these groups varied quite considerably between wards—in London, for example, physicians' assistants were mainly employed in the Medical Assessment Unit; the use of student nurses was found to differ quite significantly between wards in any given Trust; physiotherapists were more in evidence on, say, Stroke Units than other wards. Depending on where and how these groups were used, the HCA role could be shaped at the margins quite differently. For example, on some wards student nurses learning about technical tasks, squeezed out opportunities for HCAs to perform such tasks, causing some HCA frustration.

Equally significant as an influence on the shape of the HCA role was the ward's use of temporary agency staff on a shift to cover HCA or nurse shortages. Registered nurses were often much less willing to delegate tasks to these unknown and unfamiliar agency workers. (For a more detailed discussion on the impact of agency HCAs, see Chapter 8.) The consequence could be an increased burden on Trust HCAs and indeed other team members forced either to spend their time supporting the agency worker or taking on tasks that might otherwise have been performed by an experienced HCA:

> HCA_London: If a bank or agency comes in, they come in from different places, like they never work in the ward, sometimes some of them, maybe they're working in a nursing home or because of the agency, they just give them the work. They come in and they will be like so they don't know what to do, you have to show them, sometimes you find it difficult to work with them where you just have to work together and show them.

Management style

A degree of discretion in shaping the HCA role was apparent at ward level in the guise of the ward manager's style of management. Ward managers varied in how supportive they were of the HCA role and its post holders:

> HCA_London: You've got some really good members of staff over here, a couple of fantastic senior sisters that will always encourage you to go on with your knowledge and everything. But unfortunately, there are ones who say the words, 'HCA, dogsbody'.

A number of examples emerged where the ward manager's style was crucial in developing the HCA role. During observation, an instance was noted of a ward manager on a surgical ward teaching an HCA to carry out a new procedure—a bladder lavage—generating a change in the future shape of this HCA's role. Indeed there were a number of ward managers who indicated a desire to develop HCAs:

> Ward manager_North: The extended things like taking bloods and ECGs ... [HCAs] come to me and said they want to do that and I would support all of them doing it if they wanted to do it. I wouldn't push them into doing it because personally I think a Band 2, they're not paid enough for the responsibility. But if they choose to do that and that's what they want to extend their role then I'm quite happy to support that.

At the same time, there were other managers, who were less supportive of such developments:

> Matron_South: At the moment I don't want healthcare assistants doing anything that is an extended role. Purely and simply because I need to improve quality and when the HCAs are off doing obs, they're off doing bloods, they're off doing cannulation, that's what they're focusing on. I do feel quite strongly and all the HCAs and all the trained staff know it, that at the moment this is what I want my HCAs concentrating on. On an individual basis, I'm happy to discuss, you know, whether they want to go off and do a cannulation course. But I would need to be really clear and have that discussion with them that actually this wasn't going to take away from what we need them to do.

The individual

The shape of the HCA role was heavily influenced by a number of individual characteristics: disposition, capability, and personal circumstances.

Disposition

HCAs embraced the role with varying degree of commitment and enthusiasm. Some HCAs were keen to push the boundaries of the role:

> HCA_Midlands: I'm quite keen and I can do ECGs, I'm not supposed to but I can do ECGs, BMs, obs, and I used to pack the wounds, and obviously do the ordering for the ward, which for an auxiliary that's quite, not an advanced role, well no other auxiliary does it unless they've been there quite a few years. But I don't mind doing it, so I did it. But also, that helps you learn and you know everything what's needed for the ward. So when you've got these new Staff Nurses coming on the ward, they know nothing, so it's nice to teach them.

At the other end of the spectrum, there were HCAs who showed a marked reluctance to engage, at best retreating to the core of the role:

> Nurse_London: We've got another [HCA], who's on the ward and is a bit, a bit lazy, likes to sit at the desk ... You've just got to give him a bit of a kick up the bum.

The most striking example of disposition affecting the shape of the HCA role emerged in the case of the aspirational individual. These were HCAs with an ambition to develop their careers, who often sought to craft their job, taking on more tasks and seek to extend the role. It was a pattern which could cause problems on the ward with aspirational HCAs taking on more complex jobs to the neglect of core care activities:

> Nurse_South: Recently we had a healthcare assistant who was working with us and he got very keen to do cannulation and blood letting and would, 'I'll go and do that', and 'I'll look on the computer for the results' and blah, blah, blah and actually it's like you need to go and do that commode and strip that empty bed first, and you're kind of thinking, it's all very well learning these things but actually you are here to go and empty the skips and keep the trolleys stocked up, as well as do the extra role if you can.

Capability

Most obviously activities undertaken by the HCA were sensitive to the capabilities of the post holder:

> Ward manager_London: We try and treat them [HCAs] all as individuals and not every HCA is able to do everything and as much as others, so you have to value each person as an individual and you have to look at the strengths and the weaknesses on both sides.

In part, capability derived from experience. Experienced HCAs often engaged in a broad range of tasks; longevity in the role had facilitated the formal as well as on-the-job acquisition of skills and an appreciation of requisite routines:

> HCA_South: The longer you're here, the more they ask you to do, the more people will just take you aside and teach you this little thing and, 'Oh you can do that now'. It's very like that and as far as I'm concerned it's a teaching hospital, you're going to advance yourself the whole time, you're going to learn more, every situation you're put in you learn something, whether that's from something you do a hundred times.

At the same time, experience could be a double-edged sword, in certain instances narrowing the role. Older HCAs could become stuck in their ways and unwilling to venture beyond a well-established 'comfort zone':

> Nurse_South: Quite a lot of the ones who've been an HCA and are slightly on the older side, they came in to it for the patient contact and the washing and the dressing and so on, and they tend to want to stick with that, that's what they're happy doing. And if that's what they're happy with, I don't think we have to push them to do it anymore. With the younger ones, they tend to want to learn to do the observations, the blood glucose monitoring, dressings and other things. So we will teach them that and the others, we will support them in what they want to do.

Personal circumstances

The other example of job crafting arose in relation to HCAs who sought to shape the role in the context of their personal circumstances, for example, their childcare responsibilities. It has been noted that this form of crafting was most likely to be seen in bespoke patterns of working time. This took the form of only working certain shifts—say just nights—or preferring to work only long days, or only part shifts:

> HCA_London: I can't work full-time because of my family circumstances; I have to be home at certain times for my children and in the morning, you know, I can't start at like seven o'clock. So if I find a proper job which like suits my lifestyle and, you know, helps the Trust as well, then I will be happy to work, otherwise, you know, I will keep looking for it.

Types of HCA

Having relied upon the qualitative material to consider where the core of the HCA role lies and the range of factors influencing its shape, this section mainly draws on survey data. It does so as a means of exploring in a much more structured and systematic way the substantive form assumed by the role: the activities undertaken by the HCA and their configuration. The findings will be seen to confirm the malleability of the role, with tasks and activities being combined in various ways and giving rise to different types of HCA. These HCA types will be presented as partly being structurally determined, closely related to Trust and clinical division; but a residual degree of agency will also be claimed, one of the HCA types bearing the hallmarks of individual job crafting. These HCA types are characterized and an attempt is made to explain how and why they have emerged. A final mention is made about how these clusters relate to certain outcomes.

Characterization of types

Cluster analysis was performed on the survey data which asked HCAs the frequency with which different tasks were undertaken (never, daily, weekly, monthly, or annually). (A technical note on the approach adopted can be found in Kessler et al 2012a.) This analysis revealed five distinct HCA types, presented in Table 6.2.

Five types of HCA emerge from the cluster analysis. Drawing upon the conceptual distinctions set out in Chapter 1, these can be differentiated along two main dimensions: diversity—the breadth of tasks performed; and complexity—the technical sophistication of the activity undertaken. Figure 6.6 shows how the clusters are plotted against these dimensions. Each HCA type is labelled and described in turn using this two-dimensional framework to facilitate the characterization.

Cluster 1: the Bedside Technician

Cluster 1 has been labelled the 'Bedside Technician'. It is a role which revolves around the bedside provision of patient-centred direct and indirect

Table 6.2 Task frequency by HCA cluster type[a]

Task	Bedside Technician (n = 205)	Ancillary (n = 100)	Citizen (n = 132)	All Rounder (n = 38)	Expert (n = 63)	Nurses (n = 689)
Bathing	daily	weekly	daily	daily	weekly	weekly
Feeding	daily	weekly	weekly	daily	weekly	weekly
Bed making	daily	daily	daily	daily	daily	daily
Collecting TTO	monthly	weekly	daily	weekly	weekly	monthly
Escorting a patient	monthly	monthly	daily	weekly	weekly	weekly
Stocking stores	monthly	daily	daily	weekly	daily	weekly
Observations	daily	monthly	daily	daily	daily	daily
Blood monitoring	daily	yearly	daily	daily	daily	daily
Simple dressing	monthly	yearly	monthly	daily	weekly	daily
Taking blood	never	never	never	weekly	daily	monthly
Female catheterization	never	never	never	monthly	never	monthly
Complex dressing	never	never	never	monthly	never	monthly
ECG	never	never	monthly	weekly	weekly	monthly
Cannulation	never	never	never	monthly	yearly	monthly

[a] Task mean scores have been substituted with their semantic equivalent from the rating scale to ease comparison

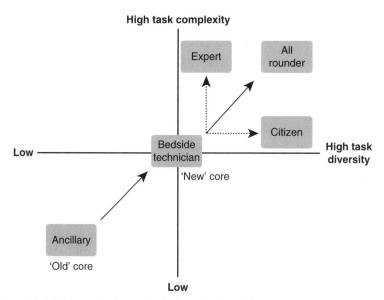

Figure 6.6 HCA types (task complexity by task diversity).

care—bathing, feeding, and bed making—which is undertaken on a daily basis. It also embraces the performance of routine technical tasks such as blood glucose monitoring (BMs) and observations, also delivered on a daily basis. This is an HCA who will carry out some other indirect care tasks including escorting patients and collecting discharge medicine (TTO)—but will never drift into the performance of more sophisticated specialist or technical tasks such as taking bloods and ECGs. Such a combination of tasks puts this HCA at the centre of our framework, performing at the mid-point in terms of complexity and diversity of tasks. It is by far the most common type of HCA, 38 per cent of individuals within our sample fell in this cluster, and consequently might legitimately be seen as today's standard HCA model.

As the standard model, it is striking that Bedside Technician not only performed direct and indirect care tasks but also undertook routine technical tasks. The role was captured in interview by an HCA falling within this type:

> HCA_South: We do our initial role, you know, care of the patients, commoding them, washing them, dressing them, feeding them, but we also do, obviously when the staff nurses are busy and maybe the bells aren't ringing, we help the nurses do the obs. We do dinners, we do blood sugars.

Taken as the new standard model, it is also worth comparing the profile of the Bedside Technician with that of the nurse. Table 6.2 confirms that while nurses continue to make beds on a daily basis, they have stepped back somewhat, if not completely, from performing other direct and indirect care tasks. The nurses' centre of gravity is the routine technical tasks of BM, observation, and simple dressings, all undertaken on a daily basis. Nurses also devote their time to the more technically sophisticated tasks such as taking bloods and cannulation, which remain essentially, if not quite exclusively, the nurses' preserve.

Cluster 2: the Ancillary HCA

Cluster 2 has been classified as the 'Ancillary'. This is an HCA who carries out only a restricted range of routine tasks—bed making and keeping stores stocked—with any frequency. It is therefore presented in the framework as a low complexity and low diversity role. While the traditional, pre-1990 'nurse auxiliary' could perform a wide range of tasks, the Ancillary HCA distinguished in our analysis appears to conform most closely to the underlying conception of this old auxiliary: supporting the ward team with the performance of fairly routine tasks, rather than acting as a regular provider of hands-on care. Nineteen per cent of HCAs fell within this cluster. It is a role reflected in the comments of an HCA interviewee:

> HCA_London: So we have a handover, then we do breakfast; most of the patients here are fed, some, a couple feed themselves, most of them now we feed or are peg-fed, so

we don't have a busy breakfast round and that's it. So we wash, get everyone washed, some people get up, most of them don't. Wash, shave, do everything for them ... and then that's it, apart from if they've dirtied the bed or something; we've got a washing machine and we tend to put the linen out.

Cluster 3: the Citizen HCA

Cluster 3 has been named the 'Citizen'. The title derives from the fact that this type of HCA is performing not only a wide range of direct and indirect care tasks on a fairly regular basis, but also tasks with a strong team orientation. For example, in contrast to the Bedside Technician, the Citizen will collect TTOs, escort patients, and in particular keep stores stocked on a daily basis. Like the Bedside Technician, the Citizen undertakes BMs and observations, while more complex technical tasks remain unfamiliar territory. This emphasis on working both for the patient and the nursing team is highlighted by this HCA:

> HCA_South: We help the nurses and we're there for the nurses. We help dish out the bowls or help the patients with a wash, make the beds. If a patient wants anything we go running, if the nurse wants us to do something we do something for them. So we are all over the place and we do a lot of work.

This combination of tasks places the Citizen HCA as high on diversity but at a mid-point on complexity. After the Bedside Technician, it is the most common type of HCA, with 25 per cent falling within this category.

Cluster 4: the All Rounder HCA

This cluster has been designated as the 'All Rounder'. It is the HCA type which works across the full range of activities. It retains the core configuration of tasks revolving around direct and indirect care, as well as retaining a focus on routine technical tasks. The level of engagement in certain team-centred tasks such as keeping stores stocked is lower than for the Citizen, but the All Rounder ventures with greater regularity into the provision of more sophisticated specialist and technical tasks. The All Rounder will therefore be taking bloods and performing ECGs with some regularity and at times even changing complex dressings. This is an HCA engaged in a highly complex and highly diverse set of tasks. It would appear to be a demanding role, the closest HCA to the nurse profile, and unsurprisingly, therefore, only a relatively small number of individuals, seven per cent, perform it. This role type is illustrated by the comments of another HCA interviewee, worth quoting at length as a means of conveying the full scale of this role:

> HCA_London: After handover we're checking probably machines or equipment. After that we're helping patients with breakfast because especially on our ward some of the

patients they need a help, they need assistance with feeding. Afterwards we're getting on with daily hygiene. We do bed baths as well and we assess skin. After that we make the patient comfortable for the day, if we can we move patients out from beds. We do observations which is the blood pressure, pulse, saturation, temperature. Of course we do all this paperwork as well, we're doing monitoring. We do observations very closely with patients when they are unstable. We check blood sugar. We help patients mobilise a lot when they likes to go to the toilet sometimes we used to go with them, that takes the time as well. I can do ECGs officially because I've done this unit as my NVQ. We do catheter care. I can catheterise females now as well. I can take bloods.

Cluster 5: the Expert HCA

Cluster 5 has been called the 'Expert'. This HCA is not as heavily engaged in certain direct and indirect care tasks, particularly bathing and feeding patients, as most of the other HCA types. The Expert type continues to perform the routine technical tasks of the other clusters but its expertise lies in an extension of the role to take on some complex technical task such as taking bloods. It does not perform as full a range of such tasks as the All Rounder but undertakes some, such as ECGs, more regularly.

> HCA_Midlands: We'll empty catheters if they need emptying. If the nurses want us to do their obs we'll do their obs, blood sugar monitoring, we'll do that, ECGs … bloods … If a patient needs escorting to X-rays, we have to go there … make sure everything's stocked up in the cupboards for like all the syringes and everything like that.

The Expert therefore scores quite highly on the complexity of tasks undertaken but performing a narrow range of such tasks, score low on diversity. A relatively small but noteworthy 12 per cent fell within this category.

In further characterizing these clusters, a fairly plausible relationship emerges between HCA type, pay banding and NVQ accreditation: the more diverse and complex the HCA type, the more likely the individual post holder is to be a Band 3 with an NVQ 3. This should not detract from the fact that complexity and diversity are not necessarily aligned with a higher banding or qualification, a consequence of HCAs being concentrated in Band 2 across all Trusts. As Table 6.3 indicates, a third of those in the most complex and diverse roles—All Rounders and Experts—were in Band 3. This clearly leaves over two-thirds of those in these most sophisticated of roles in Band 2. Predictably lower proportions of Bedside Technicians, Ancillary, and Citizen HCAs are in Band 3. Again, as might have been envisaged, the majority of All Rounders and Experts have an NVQ 3, although once more the fact that a third of All Rounders and almost a half of Experts do not have an NVQ 3 remains striking. Less surprising is the finding that only a small minority of those in the other clusters have an NVQ3.

Table 6.3 Pay band and NVQ details by cluster type (%)

	Bedside Technician	Ancillary	Citizen	All Rounder	Expert	p-value
Band 3	5	7	12	33	37	$\chi^2 = 59.80, p < 0.001$
NVQ 3	19	20	32	64	53	$\chi^2 = 51.71, p < 0.001$

Explaining types

Consideration can now be given to how and why these clusters emerge: are there patterns in the distribution of these types, and if so what explains them? Drawing on the distinction between structure and agency, a relationship between clusters and the Trust and or division would suggest the influence of structure; a relationship between HCA type and the background characteristics of the HCA—say their aspirations and length of service—might imply the significance of post holder agency.

Structure, in the form of Trust and division, emerge as significant influences on the distribution of HCA type. As Table 6.4 indicates, the profile of the four Trusts in terms of this cluster distribution is quite distinctive:

- South has a notable concentration of Ancillary HCAs: a third of its HCAs fall into this category, the highest proportion of any Trust. It also has a relatively limited proportion of its HCAs, just over quarter, in the Bedside Technician role, much lower than North and London.

- Midlands has a particularly high concentration of Citizen HCAs, over a third, markedly higher than any other Trust. Midlands is similar to the South in having a much lower proportion of Bedside Technicians than North and London but shares with North a significant group of Experts.

Table 6.4 Cluster type by Trusts (%)

	South (n = 164)	Midlands (n = 133)	North (n = 141)	London (n = 100)	p-value
Bedside Technician	29	26	55	46	
Ancillary	34	18	2	17	
Citizen	25	36	13	25	$\chi^2 = 104.79, p < 0.001$
All Rounder	9	5	9	5	
Expert	4	16	21	7	

- North has a strikingly high proportion of its HCAs as Bedside Technicians, over a half fall into this category. This is much higher than in any other Trust, although it shares a significant concentration of HCAs in this role with London. It is also a Trust with a sizeable group of Expert HCAs, close to a quarter, once more, far higher than in any other Trust.

- London shares with North an emphasis on the Bedside Technician, close to half of its HCAs falling within this category. In contrast to North, however, the other significant concentration of HCAs can be found as Citizens rather than as Experts.

Trying to understand these patterns is not easy. It is tempting to relate the relatively high concentration of Ancillary HCAs in South to the demise of the NVQ framework in that Trust: in the absence of such a framework it arguably becomes less easy for HCAs to signal their technical capabilities to nurses, perhaps encouraging them to withdraw to the most basic of tasks. Other explanations remain speculative and not immediately apparent from the systems and policies adopted by the respective Trusts. It has, after all, been suggested that Trust-wide policies and practices designed to shape the HCA role were relatively weak and permissive. There may, however, be some latent factors related to organizational culture or management style which account for this distribution of HCA types by Trust. For instance, it might be argued that the tight-knit, intimate 'everyone knows everyone' culture at Midlands accounts for the greater prevalence of 'Citizen HCAs': such a culture encouraging or reflecting a willingness amongst HCAs to 'muck-in' and contribute to the team.

The divisional distribution of HCA types is more readily explained. As Table 6.5 indicates, there is a significant difference in cluster membership across the two clinical divisions. A higher proportion of medical than surgical HCAs are likely to be Bedside Technicians: respectively close to a half compared to just over a quarter. Arguably, medical patients are more likely to be chronically dependent and somewhat older than surgical patients, requiring more intense bedside personal care. Moreover, the high proportion of Citizens in surgery might reflect the greater movement of patients on the surgical wards, and hence the greater need to escort patients, while the higher throughput of surgical patients might necessitate the more frequent collection of TTOs by HCAs.

Figure 6.7 presents significant relationships between key variables and cluster membership. The influence of individual agency on the shape of the HCA role was a key analytical tenet of our study: it has been argued that who HCAs are in terms of their background and motivation might influence how they shape their role. The survey data provided a number of plausible relationships between these kinds of factors and HCA type, although perhaps not as many as might have been expected. These are now discussed in turn.

Table 6.5 Cluster type by division (%)

	Medical (n = 364)	Surgical (n = 174)	p-value
Bedside Technician	43	28	
Ancillary	20	15	$\chi^2 = 23.80, p < 0.001$
Citizen	20	33	
All Rounder	5	12	
Expert	12	12	

Length of service

Length of service at the Trust (see Table 6.6) was related to cluster, suggesting the importance of individual tenure. The Bedside Technician, Ancillary, and Citizen HCAs were much less experienced in these terms than the All Rounder and the Expert. While around a third of Bedside Technicians, Ancillary, and Citizen HCAs had less than two years' experience, this was the case for barely 10 per cent of the All Rounders and Experts. This suggests that Trusts used the former as 'starter' roles, individuals only moving onto the latter, more diverse and complex roles, when they had built up requisite experience and skills.

Self-esteem

There was a link between self-esteem and HCA type. Self-esteem is generally conceptualized as how one regards oneself: an evaluation of personal merit

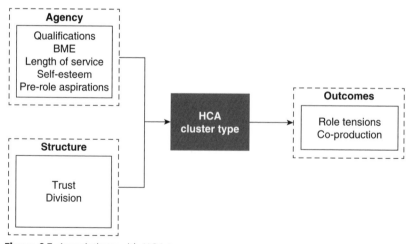

Figure 6.7 Associations with HCA types.

Table 6.6 Agency related variables by cluster type (%)

	Bedside Technician	Ancillary	Citizen	All Rounder	Expert	p-value
Less than 2 years of service	32	36	29	11	8	$\chi^2 = 36.64$, $p = 0.002$
Nurse ambitions prior to HCA role	52	37	55	63	31	$\chi^2 = 18.70$, $p = 0.001$
Self-esteem (mean score)[a]	5.11	5.25	5.27	5.32	5.39	$F = 3.65$, $p = 0.006$
Ethnicity: BME	20	23	31	18	12	$\chi^2 = 10.97$, $p = 0.027$
HCAs on ward carry out similar tasks to self	85	86	80	46	52	$\chi^2 = 56.01$, $p < 0.001$

[a] Self-enhancement subscale, measured on a six-point scale

or worth. It might feed through to influence confidence, levels of workplace performance, and the pursuit (or not) of aspirations. Self-esteem scores were high for HCAs as a group across our case study Trusts and broadly similar to those of the nurses they worked with. The relationship between self-esteem and HCA type was, however, apparent in the significantly higher levels of self-esteem reported by Experts compared to Bedside Technicians; a plausible finding given the greater confidence likely to be required when taking on more complex tasks.

Nurse aspirations

An aspiration to become a nurse on taking up the HCA role was also associated with clustering. Those with such an aspiration made up a much higher proportion of the All Rounders than any other HCA type; almost two-thirds (63%) of All Rounders had nurse ambitions, compared with barely a third of Expert and Ancillary HCAs. Again this is a correlation which might readily be explained by the HCAs' search for experience and new capabilities in pursuit of their aspirations.

Ethnicity

There was a connection between ethnicity and cluster. The Citizen type comprised a markedly higher proportion of those with a BME background than other clusters: almost a third (31%) of this cluster type had an ethnic background compared to 12 per cent of Experts. Some care is needed in generalizing to suggest that the cultures of those with BME backgrounds lend themselves more to a communal, team spirit. Nonetheless, there might well be differences in ethnic values which account for this finding.

Role shaping

Finally, a couple of further pieces of evidence suggested the residual importance of post holder agency. The first emerged when drilling down into the distribution of HCA types by ward and more discrete clinical areas: such an analysis revealed that while small in number, the All Rounder HCA is found across a wider range of wards and areas than the Citizen and Expert, who are confined to particular clinical spheres. The All Rounder appears to be unconstrained and undeterred by structural factors associated with ward or area. This is confirmed by a second piece of survey evidence which finds a relatively low proportion of All Rounders claiming that 'HCAs are doing the same things on their ward': under a half (46%) of All Rounders note that HCAs on their ward carry out the same range of tasks, while the figure is over 80 per cent for the Beside Technician, Ancillary, and Citizen HCAs. The All Rounder emerges as a maverick, breaking free from structural determinants by shaping a different role on the ward to that of her or his colleagues.

Types and outcomes

While the next chapters deal in detail with the consequences of the HCA role for various stakeholders, it is briefly worth exploring whether these different types of HCA were associated with any outcome variables in the survey. The survey revealed some striking and plausible relationships. All Rounders were significantly more likely to perceive role tensions with nurses than Ancillary HCAs, unsurprising given that the former rather than latter were pushing at role boundaries. Moreover, the Citizen HCA scored significantly higher on co-production than the Bedside Technician. This is perhaps less easy to explain, given that co-production related in part to care tasks: it might, however, reflect the greater ability of an HCA performing non-care tasks for the patient to contribute in a distinctive way.

Notwithstanding these findings, stronger links with outcome variables might have been expected. One might reasonably have assumed a significant relationship between HCA type and job satisfaction: for example, the diversity of the All Rounder role might lead to greater job satisfaction than amongst other types of HCA, with scope to push the boundaries of the role; by the same token the Ancillary might have been expected to more dissatisfied in finding their role confined to more routine tasks. The absence of such links suggests future lines of analysis. First, there might well be grounds for the absence of such a link: for instance, All Rounders might have had higher expectations for the role, with the ability to shape it as desired not reflected in higher satisfaction but a cognitive acknowledgement that this was no more or less than envisaged. Second, and closely related, the weak link between HCA type and outcomes encourages the search for more refined measures allowing the relationship to be further explored: measures perhaps related to the personality and orientation of the individual to their role and additional attitudinal and behavioural outcomes. Third, the relationship between HCA type and these sorts of outcomes might be moderated by various factors weakening any assumed link: for example, the high job satisfaction of those in routine roles might well reflect benefits from the role beyond the tasks performed, such as convenient working hours. In turning more fully to the consequences of the HCA role in the following chapters, the analysis moves away from HCA types to the presentation of findings which more generally relate to impact.

Summary

The purpose of this chapter was to look behind the generic job title to explore more precisely the shape and nature of the HCA role. The open and incomplete nature of the employment relationship suggests that any broadly conceived job title is unlikely to capture the diverse forms assumed by the enacted work role. The evolution of the HCA role over many years, as captured by myriad occupational labels, pointed to the likelihood of an unusually varied and complex configuration of tasks and responsibilities. The picture to emerge from this chapter not only highlights the malleable nature of a HCA role, sensitive to a range of factors, but more precisely delineates different role types and relates them to the interplay between structure and agency.

The chapter was divided into three parts. The first searched for the core of the HCA role. Drawing upon the qualitative data, that which related to perceptions of who the HCA supported and what made a 'good' HCA, it was apparent that the views of the various stakeholders differed: in broad terms, HCAs had more of a patient-centric view of the role; nurses, a nurse-centric perspective, and ward managers, a team-centric outlook. However, there was a general consensus that the HCA role centred on the delivery of direct patient care, and at the same time had the capacity to extend and take on a broader range of ward-based and technical tasks.

The capacity of the HCA role to assume different forms encouraged a grounded search for contingent influential factors. The second section focused on these contingent influences and revealed the importance of four sets of factors associated with: Trust-wide policies and practices; the clinical area; the ward; and the individual post holder. Building upon these findings it was possible to develop a survey instrument and undertake cluster analysis on the frequency with which a range of tasks were performed. This uncovered five types of HCA role: the Ancillary, the Bedside Technician, the Citizen, the All Rounder, and the Expert.

These role types were found to vary according to the diversity and the complexity of the tasks performed. Moreover, the incidence of these types was plausibly related to structure—the Trust and clinical area—and to agency— job crafting by the individual post holder. Despite the presence of these different roles, most striking was confirmation that the standard type of HCA, the Bedside Technician, along with some other HCA types, was providing not only direct patient care but also routinely undertaking low-level technical tasks. Certainly the contemporary HCA role had moved a long way since its original conception as an auxiliary, hands-off support.

The findings were less conclusive on the impact of these different HCA types on various outcomes, such as job satisfaction. However, a major component of the research focused on the consequences of the HCA role for different stakeholders, and it is to this component that attention now turns.

Issues for reflection

The findings in this chapter suggest the need for Trusts to consider:

- The different perceptions of who the HCA is supporting and what makes a 'good' HCA held by ward team members.
- Whether these perceptions accord with and are anchored in current job descriptions and person specifications for the HCA role.
- The different influences on the shape of the HCA role—Trust, ward, division, and individual—and how these might be more explicitly leveraged to design the role in desired ways.
- The particular importance of influences at ward level on the HCA role: for example, ward manager style and capability, the deployment of student nurses, and the patterns of work organization.
- The different forms assumed by the HCA role, especially the five HCA types distinguished. Assessment could be made of the following: how and why these types are distributed in particular ways within the Trust; whether this distribution is in line with the intended HCA contribution at the Trust; how these types might be used as the basis for a more refined form of workforce and skill mix planning.

Chapter 7

Consequences for healthcare assistants

HCA_North: I've wanted this [HCA job] for so, so long and never been able to do it. I applied at another hospital eleven times and they just never got back in touch with me. And now I'm here. It's just so interesting and I just love it; compared to supermarket work, it's absolutely wonderful, I love it.

HCA_South: I don't think we're respected much: you quite often hear people go 'oh she's only an HCA' or 'oh that's an HCA's job', and that's a little bit degrading.

Introduction

It will be recalled that the impact of the HCA role on those groups with a stake in it was presented in terms of positive and negative scenarios. These were not necessarily mutually exclusive to one another, the role potentially affecting these stakeholders in contradictory or ambiguous ways. For HCAs themselves, the role might create a degraded ghetto and/or provide an opportunity for a more enriching working life. For nurses, the HCA role might lend valuable support and or bring with it new burdens and uncertainties. For patients, the HCA might represent a more accessible, less intimidating source of care and/ or may raise doubts about care quality and bring with it certain perceived risks. The next three chapters of the book will consider the outcomes of the HCA role respectively for the three main stakeholders in these terms, seeking to establish whether or how the positive and negative combine. This chapter focuses on HCAs, and the succeeding chapters, in turn, on nurses and patients.

In exploring outcomes for the HCAs themselves, a number of criteria were used:

- The management of HCAs;
- The fulfilment of HCA aspirations and career intentions;
- HCA general 'likes' and 'dislikes' and more precisely job satisfaction and intention to leave;
- The emotional intensity of the role for HCAs.

The picture to emerge suggests that across our Trusts, and with some variation between them, the consequences of the HCA role for post holders are often emotionally intense and not always positive, particularly in the context of the effort–reward bargain and relations with nurses and other professionals. However, in general, HCAs display a strong attachment to and enjoyment of their jobs, a finding reflected in high levels of job satisfaction and low intention to quit.

The management of HCAs

The management of HCAs, as assessed by Trust approaches to HCA induction, training, performance management, voice, and pay and grading showed signs of unevenness. However, there were some common, cross cutting patterns. Indeed, there are grounds for arguing that in important respects the management of HCAs was underdeveloped across Trusts, to the point where questions of 'fairness' emerged.

Induction

In all four Trusts induction was characterized by a common core, which revolved around a corporate introduction to all new starters across the Trust, followed by some additional mandatory training days and an extended period of a week or two shadowing a member of the team at ward level. Although HCAs typically felt well enough prepared to take on the role, HCA induction did vary between Trusts. For example, London devoted a number of dedicated days to HCA induction at corporate level, covering such topics as last offices, which was not found elsewhere.

Most HCAs felt that they were sufficiently prepared to perform the role from the outset, with shadowing of team members being viewed as especially useful. Indeed, it was clear that for many HCAs this on-the-job phase of induction was critical to learning about the details of the role:

> HCA_North: It was sufficient because we'd been on the ward supernumerary for two weeks before we went for the induction; because there was obviously so many that

were starting at different times; they had to put us all through at the same time for the induction. So mainly we'd learnt a lot off the nurses and the other healthcares on the ward when we came here and first started.

There were, however, some concerns about preparation for the role. In Midlands with just three days' corporate induction, one HCA noted:

> HCA_Midlands: I was thrown in to it. They don't give you enough time. I think they'll put you on a one or two day induction and they think 'oh right, she's OK'. I mean we've got two girls on our ward who have just been thrown in really, and they hadn't come from the nursing backgrounds so they haven't got a clue.

Induction sessions in the different trusts were often held at set intervals, and so many times of year. In London this was found to delay HCA recruitment which needed to coincide with an induction. In North, recruitment went ahead regardless of a scheduled induction, the result being that some HCAs were in post without having attended a corporate induction.

Training

At the time of the research, the main form of training for HCAs resided in the application of the NVQ framework. However, its use was markedly uneven between the four Trusts, with some quite dramatic differences in the proportion of HCAs holding NVQ qualifications. As Table 7.1 indicates, South had relatively few HCAs with either NVQ 2 (23%) or NVQ 3 (17%), and even those who had acquired these qualifications were unlikely to have done so at the Trust (37%). In contrast, almost three quarters of HCAs at London had an NVQ level 2, two-thirds receiving it whilst at the Trust. Equally striking is the fact that over half of the HCAs at Midlands had a NVQ 3, 'out-performing' London in this respect.

Table 7.1 Pay bands and NVQ qualifications (%)

	South	Midlands	North	London	p-value
Band 2[a]	80	82	90	82	$\chi^2 = 8.69, p = 0.034$
Band 3	18	18	8	16	
NVQ level 1	9	12	11	21	$\chi^2 = 8.37, p = 0.039$
NVQ level 2	23	58	43	70	$\chi^2 = 67.12, p < 0.001$
NVQ level 3	17	51	22	30	$\chi^2 = 49.36, p < 0.001$
NVQ attained at this Trust	37	58	57	69	$\chi^2 = 14.93, p = 0.002$

[a] Band 1 (n = 9) and Band 4 (n = 1) have been omitted from this table

There were also some generic problems cutting across the Trusts with the model of NVQ accreditation. In part these were operational difficulties: a number of Trusts had difficulty finding enough NVQ assessors, whilst with understaffing on the ward, HCAs could face problems in finding time to attend designated teaching sessions. These work pressures were sometimes combined with personal difficulties in engaging with NVQ training, ranging from non-work constraints to the intimidating nature of a formal learning situation for some:

> HCA_London: [Acquiring an NVQ is] very intense and quite hard-going. I'm a full-time mum, I've got a house to run and to try and study, I find it quite hard because it's like eleven o'clock at night before I can sit there and try and get my work out and then trying to concentrate when you're tired, you've been up since six, it's quite tough.

However, the marked differences between Trusts in the level of HCA accreditation can be explained by contrasting approaches to the application of NVQ framework between the respective organizations. Three such approaches were distinguished. First, and accounting for its low level of accreditation, South had effectively allowed their NVQ infrastructure to 'wither on the vine':

> Manager_South: A lot of Trusts have strong support for NVQs ... So they'll say, 'Oh the government expects 80 per cent of the workforce to have NVQ level 3 so let's do something about it' ... but our Trust realised, 'well if we don't do anything about it nobody's going to bother to chase this up, so let's ignore this one' ... So I think a lot of Trusts do put their support around NVQs and then they'll have quite a few study days associated with that ... Our solution is very different, it's let's write our own which are much more accessible for staff, maintain competence and a structure to the development but don't tie people up in bureaucracy and paperwork like NVQs.

Second, North had retained a commitment to the NVQ model, but its approach was reactive and opportunistic:

> Senior manager_North: We have an NVQ centre that functions within the organisation but, again, there's no consistency across the organisation in terms of being able to say that absolutely every support worker has gone through that. (It) also connects with the Band 3 support workers; it's about staff at that level. If we've got people working at Band 3 then they've undertaken the NVQ 3; I think it is less robust for support workers working at level 2.

Third, in London and Midlands a much more proactive approach to NVQs was in evidence, reflected in the higher levels of accreditation. London, for example, was a centre for NVQ accreditation and had displayed some innovation in providing online access to NVQ modular material:

> Manager_London: They [HCAs] are all offered NVQ level 2 or level 3 and there is an expectation within the Trust that all healthcare assistants within [London] should have a level 2 or level 3 and it's in like their job descriptions.

Beyond the NVQ framework, HCA training opportunities were more limited. Certainly, Trusts were beginning to develop more dedicated training for HCAs. As a matron at North noted:

> Matron_North: We're getting better as a Trust. A lot of things like the infection control stuff was always directed at qualified nurses, they've now the separate courses for non-qualified and including ward clerks and things. Obviously there's the short courses; the day courses around cannulation, phlebotomy, all that that never used to be open to healthcares. We do bereavement counselling courses for healthcares, so there's a lot of things that were accessible for qualified staff they've now tailored for the healthcares as well.

As implied, these were, however recent developments. Indeed, there were concerns in Trusts at the lack of dedicated training beyond NVQs for HCAs:

> Nurse_Midlands: The auxiliary training is tending to be just mandatory and anything new that they're introducing, there might be a study day on it, but that tends to be for everyone, not just auxiliaries.
>
> HCA_London: We [HCAs] do go to the basic life support trainings whenever the ward can allow us and also fire training when the ward can allow us. We're a very busy unit, we have always been busy. But it would have been nice if they had allowed us to have more training off the ward, on the ward, it doesn't matter, even fifteen minutes' training on the ward would be great.

Performance appraisal

The disordered relationship between HCA capability and banding was not helped by the patchy application of performance management across the Trusts. With the KSF still settling down in all four Trusts, responsibility for the associated Performance Development Reviews (PDRs) was often delegated to Band 6 nurses looking after a team of HCAs for this and other management purposes. However, the extent to which PDRs were completed varied from ward to ward within the same Trust, completion being sensitive to such factors as ward manager style and perceived pressures on the ward. So in the London Trust there was a ward manager who had successfully completed all PDRs for HCAs:

> Ward manager_London: We've got it sussed, well we've got it sussed now. We do them all in sort of November/December time, they're full appraisals. At the moment we're doing their mid-term PDRs to make sure that we're getting through the training and things. Everybody has their own folder which they make their portfolio out of now, and with things that they've done, they put it in their folder so they can show us and it's something to be proud of really.

While elsewhere in the same Trust there were HCAs who had been let down by the process:

> Ward manager_London: I try [to do PDRs] but it's very, very difficult because we're so busy and manic, and every time we try and do it something happens.

The uneven completion of PDRs was disappointing given that HCAs exposed to the process were often positive about it:

> HCA_London: It [the PDR] can be quite good actually. Because I think sometimes you can get quite complacent in a job and it is nice to say well, you need to sort of shuffle your shoes a bit in that area or if you're not doing well in that area, sort of have a little directional push. Because sometimes I think you can get complacent and don't even know yourself; so I think sometimes that sort of thing is good.
>
> HCA_South: It's nice to hear some feedback on how we're all doing, it's one of the those things you think you're going to hear bad feedback but they'd let you know, as you're going they'd stop you straight away and say you don't do that, that's wrong.

Voice

The positive orientation amongst HCAs to PDRs might reflect the opportunity it provided for a form of direct voice: the chance to talk to and receive views from the ward manager or a senior nurse. It was an opportunity particularly valuable given the underdeveloped nature of other forms of HCA voice across all Trusts. HCA voice might be considered in a number of ways: as a direct or unmediated individual or collective voice expressed at ward, divisional or Trust level; or as an indirect voice articulated and expressed by and through a third party (union) representative. It is an important distinction, but in both senses HCA voice was fairly weak.

While there were forums at Trust level where HCAs could express a direct individual voice, for example, Midlands had a regular, open staff forum, this voice was most likely to be heard at ward level. In general, ward systems of staff engagement were inclusive, with HCAs routinely present at handovers at the beginning of the shift, and invited to regular ward team meetings as well as clinical days. How confident HCAs were in expressing their views at these meetings is more open to debate. On the shifts observed, HCAs were rarely seen as making an input into handover. Indeed, more generally HCAs were perhaps daunted by the prospect of contributing to ward meetings involving professionals:

> HCA_London: It's only me and another girl, we went to the ward meeting, and there was only two qualified and us two HCAs and we weren't sure if we should have said anything afterwards because you're supposed to bring up stuff and … You know, we both sort of looked at each other and thought, 'Oh alright, maybe we shouldn't have spoken', but we were just, you know, saying what we thought. There was a couple of things we brought up and, and sort of we got like shot down, and we sort of looked at each other and thought, 'Well aren't we supposed to say', you know, or, 'Maybe next time we won't say anything then, you know, if that's the case'.

Most striking was the absence of any form of direct collective HCA voice. Across the four Trusts it was difficult to find any form of dedicated meeting which allowed HCAs to convene as a group, to articulate and to express their views whether at Trust, division, or ward level: on only two wards across the four Trusts covered was any attempt made to convene HCA meetings. This might well reflect competing views on the value of a dedicated HCA forum, well articulated by a manager in London:

> Manager_London: They [HCAs] don't have a separate voice and in fact very recently we've had conversations about establishing a forum for HCAs and maybe an annual event, if nothing else, whereby they can get together and present their work and talk about their challenges and just really have an audience with people. There's a counter-argument to that though that if you're hiving them off to be seen as being separate, and maybe you should actually keep them in with nursing and midwifery, in the general body of it.

The general absence of an effective, direct HCA voice was hardly compensated by a strong representative voice. The survey revealed some striking differences in union membership between our Trusts (see Table 7.2): in Midlands almost three-quarters of the HCAs were in a union, whereas in the other three Trusts membership stayed well below a half and in South remained at a quarter. Despite these differences in density, the union organization at all Trusts remained fragile. Each had a joint consultative or negotiation committee covering all non-medical staff at Trust level, but the individual HCAs' connection to such machinery was tenuous. As a ward manager in North noted:

> Ward manager_North: I'm on a lot of disciplinary panels and things like that and I would say [HCAs] are a group of people who are very poorly represented because they don't actually have any membership of any kind of unions or anything and they're not quite sure of the right direction. I mean nurses are always well represented by the RCN, but they're [HCAs] poorly represented and often come on their own. So I suppose from that point of view they obviously don't get the right support.

In large part this lack of individual connection with the union was a consequence of weak forms of ward representation in the Trusts; there were very few HCA union representatives in any of the hospitals; such representatives were simply not a meaningful presence at ward level. Indeed, in Midlands, the Trust with the highest union density, only four out of ten interviewed HCAs who were union members knew the name of their local lay representative.

Table 7.2 Union membership (%)

	South	Midlands	North	London	p-value
Union member	25	70	44	37	$\chi^2 = 69.01, p < 0.001$

Pay and grading

The management of HCA pay and grading raises some fundamental questions about the treatment of post holders. In all four Trusts, the HCA workforce was overwhelmingly concentrated in Band 2. As Table 7.1 indicates, in three cases around 80 per cent of HCAs were at Band 2, while in the fourth—North—almost all HCAs were in this band. Despite the availability of a Band 3 level, clearly it was very rarely used by our Trusts. Such a compression of HCAs into Band 2 raises doubts about the effective use of pay both to support and reflect the performance and capability of HCAs. Indeed, the shortcomings of pay banding in these respects raises broader issues related to 'fairness' in the management of HCAs.

'Fairness' has been conceptualized and interpreted in very different ways. For the purposes of this discussion, it might simply be viewed as related to the alignment between three factors:

- pay band;
- qualification; and
- the diversity/complexity of the role (see Figure 7.1).

The alignment between these three aspects of employment is crucial to any assessment of fair treatment. Table 7.3 presents a series of fair and unfair combinations between the three factors:

Fair combinations:

- Band 2 and 3 roles might be seen as fairly treated if aligned respectively with NVQ levels 2 (Fi) and 3 (Fiii): in these cases HCA have the appropriate

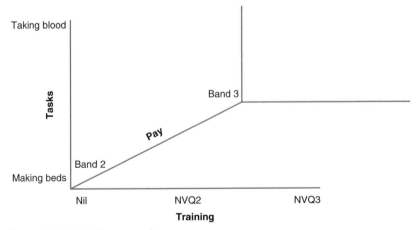

Figure 7.1 HCA effort–reward nexus.

qualifications for their band. By the same token fair treatment might be associated with Band 2s in a lower diversity/complexity role (Fii) and Band 3s in a higher diversity/complexity role (Fiv).

Unfair combinations:

- Band 2 HCAs are unfairly treated if post holders have an NVQ3 (Ui): this might be seen as the HCA being 'over-qualified' given their band. Unfairness might also arise where the HCA is undertaking a high diversity/complexity job (Uii): a case of the HCA 'over-performing' given their band.

- At the same time, those in Band 3 roles might be unfairly treated if they have an NVQ 2 (Uiii)—in essence they are 'under qualified' for the band—or if they have a low diversity/complexity job (Uiv): a case of 'under-performing' given the band level.

Given the limited use of Band 3 in our Trusts, issues of fairness or unfairness at this level were not particularly pervasive. In general, it was rare for Band 3 HCAs not to be at the appropriate NQV3. It was not, however, unknown. Thus, there were instances of unfairness at this level in the sense that Band 3 HCAs were under qualified: across the three Trusts (Midlands, North, and London) with a viable NVQ system in place, almost a quarter of Band 3s did not have an NVQ3. One HCA explained how she found herself in this situation: gaining a Band 3 on the basis of experience, rather than qualification.

> HCA_South: One or two people weren't happy that I was put up to Band 3 without achieving my NVQ, I've got it all on my experience and what I can do.
> Matron_London: I mean I would say … because of previous management we've got Band 3s in the department that haven't even got an NVQ. That's just what they were given at the time when they were taken on.

Given the compression of HCAs into the lower grade in Trusts, any unfairness is more likely to lie at Band 2 level. Indeed, instances of over qualification are highlighted in Table 7.1 with Band 2 HCAs often having an NVQ 3. This was particularly marked in Midlands, with its high proportion of NVQ 3s, and to a lesser but still significant extent in London.

Table 7.3 Fairness combinations

Unfair (U)	Fair (F)
i) Band 2—NVQ 3	i) Band 2—NVQ 2
ii) Band 2—Task diversity/complexity (high)	ii) Band 2—Task diversity/complexity (low)
iii) Band 3—NVQ 2	iii) Band 3—NVQ 3
iv) Band 3—Task diversity/complexity (low)	iv) Band 3—Task diversity/complexity (high)

Over performing also appeared to be prevalent, with many examples of HCAs in extended roles at band 2:

> Interviewer: So although you've gone back to Band 2 from Band 3, you haven't changed what you do at all?
>
> HCA_Midlands: No, in fact I'm doing a lot more. They (nurses) know you'll do it, you know so, they're unfair; they put more on to you. If your staff nurses are good to you, so be it, but I think I am doing a lot more, you know, I think the only thing I'm not probably doing is drugs and drug rounds, everything else I'm doing as a staff nurse role.
>
> HCA_Midlands: We do the ECGs, the blood pressures, the monitoring of patients, that kind of thing, whereas normally in the hospital you'd be a Band 3 [sic], but [here on this ward] you're a 2.
>
> Ward manager_North: We'd looked at skilling some [HCAs] up to Band 3s and to be honest some of them do bloods and do ECGs now but the Trust still just pays them Band 2s.
>
> Manager_London: I'm sure you will find Band 2s putting cannulae in or taking blood. I'm aware of issues such as the Band 2s' salary and it does make me think, is it fair to expect somebody to take on those kinds of roles and does it feel a bit like some sort of exploitation?

This pattern of unfair treatment, with Band 2 HCAs over-qualified or over-performing, can be viewed in a number of ways. Over-qualification—Band 2 HCAs with an NVQ3—might well encourage the withholding of extended capabilities developed through training. Such outcomes raise managerial concerns about the wasted time and cost associated with training HCAs to NVQ3 level, and about the unused capacity within the workforce. There were signs of such withholding of capabilities by HCAs, predictably in Midlands with its turmoil over skill mix (see earlier):

> HCA_Midlands: You don't want to do it [undertake an extended HCA role]; you think well why should I, if somebody's getting the recognition for it, you know getting Band 3 and the pay, reward for it and we've got to do it at Band 2, where is it justified?
>
> HCA_Midlands: As a Band 2 I think a lot of people stick to their job role.
>
> Matron_Midlands: The staff have just crawled back in their shell now and thought actually I don't know what's coming round the corner, I'll just do my basic Band 2.

Indeed, this response was also reflected in survey data which suggested (see Table 7.4) that HCAs in all Trusts felt they had the ability to carry out more complex tasks than they currently undertook.

The instances of HCA over-performance, with Bands 2s engaging in extended activities, might be viewed in a more straightforward sense as 'cheap labour'. Clearly the Trust is extracting more from their HCAs at this level, than their pay banding would suggest they were entitled.

Table 7.4 Propensity to extend the role (mean score)

	South	Midlands	North	London	p-value
My potential is not fully realized in my current role[a]	3.59	3.61	3.58	3.32	$F = 1.52$, $p = 0.208$
I believe that I have the ability to successfully carry out more complex tasks than I am currently doing	4.20	4.17	4.30	4.16	$F = 0.84$, $p = 0.474$
I have enough to do in my current role without taking on more complex tasks[a]	2.53	2.77	2.77	2.93	$F = 2.60$, $p = 0.051$
I am always looking for ways to extend my role	4.10	4.01	3.96	4.06	$F = 0.61$, $p = 0.607$
SCALE: Propensity to extend	**3.84**	**3.74**	**3.76**	**3.66**	$F = 1.33$, $p = 0.265$

[a] Scoring reversed when item included in the scale

Aspirations and career intentions

One of the clearest indicators of whether the HCA role had a negative impact on the working lives of post holders was the extent to which it provided a meaningful basis for the pursuit of career aspirations. The general data on this question were somewhat ambiguous. As Figure 7.2 indicates, there was moderate agreement across the four Trusts to the suggestion that 'there are career opportunities for [HCAs] at the Trust': over half (54%) of the HCAs 'agreed' or 'strongly agreed' with this statement. However, the response to the suggestion that their 'potential was not fully realized' were at a similar level, again over half (55%) 'agreed' or 'strongly agreed' with the assertion. It is a picture which suggests that in an abstract sense HCAs felt they had chances to develop their careers, but in personal terms, taking advantage of these chances was perhaps more problematic and difficult.

A consideration of career intentions provides a clearer picture. Such intentions were reviewed in terms of whether the HCA was seeking to: develop within the HCA role, acquiring more capabilities and become a 'high performing' HCA; use the HCA role as a stepping-stone to become a registered nurse; or deploy it as a bridge to another profession or a job outside health and social care.

The delineation of this clear set of future options should not detract from the uncertainties informing HCA career plans:

> HCA_London: I don't know exactly because I really want to do the nursing but I don't know yet. I'm just thinking about what are my family commitments, because

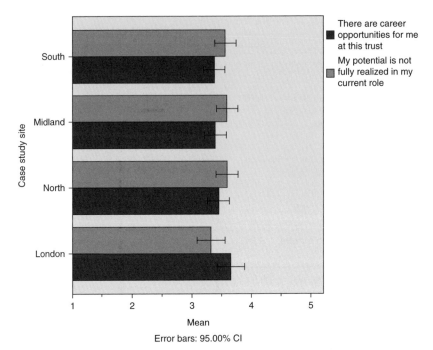

Figure 7.2 Career opportunities and realization of potential (mean).

I've got two young children at the moment and it's because of them I'm doing part-time work
HCA_North: I don't know [whether I want to be a nurse]. I mean I do, it keeps popping in to me head and like I say, when I see them all stressed out like that I think no, but then I think no, you can do that. I talk myself in and out of it, to be honest.

Notwithstanding these uncertainties, Table 7.5, presenting survey data on HCA aspirations, suggests a fairly similar pattern in three of the Trusts (South, Midlands, and North): around half of the HCAs see themselves continuing in

Table 7.5 Aspirations of HCAs (%)

In the future I want to:	South	Midlands	North	London	p-value
Continue in current job	56	61	48	45	
Train to be a registered nurse	27	26	26	40	
Train to be an allied health/social care professional	9	4	9	2	$\chi^2 = 29.30$,
Leave for job outside of health/ social care	4	3	4	7	$p = 0.004$
Other	4	7	13	5	

the role and around a quarter assume a move into registered nursing. In London, a significantly higher proportion (40%) of HCAs regard their future in terms of registered nursing, a finding which might be related to the relatively strong NVQ training culture at this Trust, and the career pathways that this established.

Amongst those who viewed their future in terms of staying as HCAs, there were some who were content to 'tread water' by continuing to routinely perform established tasks and with little commitment to in-role progression:

> Ward manager_North: None of the ones [HCAs] that have been here a while have shown any interest in sort of further developing professionally, and sometimes it might be a case of they come to work, they do what they've got to do and they go home, and if they think they're being pushed too much to do something they will say, and they will have a bit of a moan about it.

However, other HCAs were keen to develop within the role. This is illustrated in South where the degeneration of the NVQ infrastructure had not deterred some HCAs from acquiring new capabilities:

> Ward manager_South: Recently, because some of the HCAs have not been given as much opportunity to do the NVQ 3; the Trust can't financially afford it so it's a very, very selective procedure and only a very few number every year are allowed to do it. So the HCAs are taking it upon themselves to do courses internally that will allow them to progress without necessarily doing the NVQ 3 per se.

A similar view on the enthusiasm of HCAs to develop in-role was expressed in Midlands:

> Nurse_Midlands: We've got a few that are less experienced but the majority of our auxiliaries are fairly experienced and they're also very keen to learn, not just in terms of tasks but learn what goes behind those tasks and have the knowledge behind what they're doing.

Harder evidence on the willingness of HCAs to develop in the role is provided by the HCA survey, and particularly by HCA propensity to extend their role (see Table 7.5). As Figure 7.3 indicates, the average mean score on this scale amongst those who saw their future in the HCA role was moderately high, although it is striking that increasing length of service progressively dulled propensity to extend, significantly so for those with 20 or more years compared to those with two years or less service.

A number of reasons emerged to explain why the majority did not see the HCA role as a stepping-stone to registered nursing. Some HCAs enjoyed their current job so much that they did not want to become a nurse:

> HCA_North: I'm quite happy to do what I'm doing because as far as I'm concerned I do just as much as they do and I think I'm valued just as much as they are. If we weren't they wouldn't have us, would they?

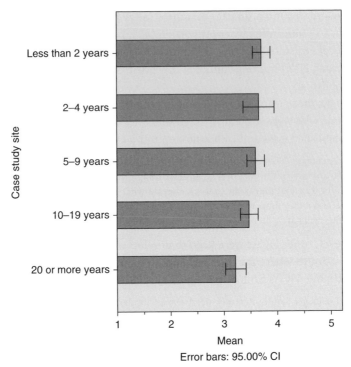

Figure 7.3 Propensity to extend the role by length of service (mean).

For others, working closely with the registered nurses had brought home some of the 'downsides' of registered nursing, discouraging any move into it:

> HCA_South: Because I see all the crap and stress they [nurses] have to go through and all the responsibility and at the end of the day everything falls on their shoulders if they've done something wrong, and that is a hell of a lot to take and I really don't think I'd want that.

More significantly, there were a number of perceived barriers facing HCAs wishing to make the move into registered nursing:

- Lack of confidence:
> HCA_Midlands: I don't see myself as confident enough to do something like that it's a big responsibility at the end of the day, give the nurses their due ... I'm quite happy having all the patient contact really.
> HCA_South: Well I would like to do my nursing, now I've been here like four and a half years I'd love to do it, but I'm not confident enough to go for it. But that would be nice, that would be an idea.

- Too old:
> HCA_Midlands: I wish I had done it [nursing] actually but, you know, it's three years and I'm fifty-five now and I think well, perhaps if I'd have done it when I first came here I'd of felt different.

- Domestic and financial pressures:

  HCA_London: I would love to do my nurse training but the way that I look at it is that I'd like to be seconded to that, purely because I can't afford to become a student. I'm a working mum, my son's doing his A levels, as you know houses are hard enough to keep above water nowadays.

For those who saw their future in registered nursing, the enduring nature of this ambition was particularly noteworthy. As Figure 7.4 indicates, there was little attrition of ambition with length of service: for those with up to nine years service well over half of them retained the ambition to be a nurse. It was only when HCAs had been in post for ten or more years that this 'dream' began to wane significantly. There is some poignancy in this picture, with deeply embedded nurse ambitions only displaced after perhaps many years of disappointment.

Likes and dislikes

The problems highlighted in managing HCAs and some of the uncertainties and ambiguities revealed about career opportunities did not feed into general

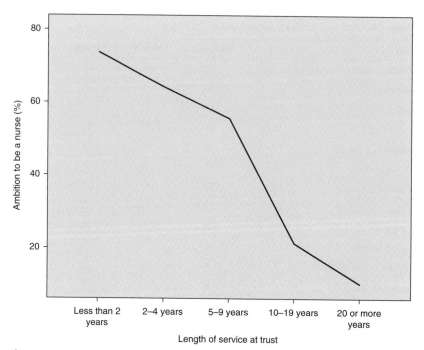

Figure 7.4 Current ambition to be a nurse by length of service. (Base: HCAs who entered the role with nurse ambitions (n = 252)).

views on the attractiveness of the HCA role. In broad terms, HCAs greatly enjoyed their jobs; indeed when asked about their 'likes' and 'dislikes', some had difficulty identifying any dislikes:

> HCA_North: I enjoy my job. I enjoy most of it, there's not anything I can particularly say that I dislike about it.
> HCA_London: I do enjoy my job, that's why I'm working here and I manage my life with two small kids and full-time work because I want to do it, otherwise I just would resign.

Most of the 'likes' identified were patient-centred, revolving around the intrinsic reward associated with caring for others and 'making a difference':

> HCA_Midlands: I enjoy my patients, patients' relatives and I talk to them. I enjoy talking with them. And I meet people, I enjoy it, and I meet different, different people.
> HCA_London: When I give my best care to the patient and when the patient then says, 'Oh thank you love, thank you'. I enjoy it, I know I've done my best. I have done something for that patient, especially when they appreciate it, and sometimes they will even say some of the staff are very good so I enjoy that.

These patient-centred 'likes' were confirmed in the survey. As Table 7.6 indicates, by far the most enjoyable tasks are related to direct and sustained patient

Table 7.6 Most enjoyable HCA tasks (HCAs: %)[a]

Task	South	Midlands	North	London	Total
Bathing	51	29	52	41	52
Feeding	47	28	29	38	41
Bed making	19	13	27	12	20
Collecting TTO	8	14	10	11	7
Escorting a patient	17	28	19	27	18
Stocking stores	6	17	4	8	6
Observations	40	52	42	52	46
Blood monitoring	27	21	19	23	24
Simple dressing	28	28	30	24	28
Taking blood	10	20	17	14	12
Female catheterization	5	1	4	7	5
Complex dressing	7	6	8	3	6
ECG	15	22	18	18	17
Cannulation	11	1	9	4	6

[a] Table figures refer to the percentage of HCAs that selected each task as one of their three choices and therefore figures will not sum to 100%

contact: the most commonly enjoyable task was bathing patients, mentioned by over half of respondents (52%), followed by feeding patients (42%).

This enjoyment of the role was also reflected in general levels of job satisfaction and intention to leave. As can be seen from Table 7.7, with the exception of pay, the mean scores on aspects of their treatment are above the mid-point, in some cases considerably so, in all Trusts. Indeed on the strongest indicator of intention to leave—leaving as soon as another job is found—mean scores in all hospital are very low, suggesting little serious propensity to quit (see Table 7.8).

This generally positive view of the role should not, however, detract from concerns raised by HCAs about their working lives, often related to relations with nurses and other professions, as well as to their institutional treatment.

The concerns around the job often related to relationships with other professional groups, in particular doctors and more importantly registered nurses. For most HCAs, contact with doctors was rare and fleeting:

HCA_Midlands: I find doctors don't talk a lot, do they.
HCA_South: I think in the time I've been here I've probably had about four or five conversations with doctors, most of them see past us, we just don't [talk to them].

Table 7.7 Job satisfaction (mean score)

	South	Midlands	North	London	p-value
The recognition I get for good work	3.37	3.13	3.34	3.10	$F = 1.98$, $p = 0.115$
The support I get from my immediate manager	3.72	3.52	3.66	3.51	$F = 1.14$, $p = 0.331$
The freedom I have to choose my own method of working	3.67	3.58	3.70	3.55	$F = 0.78$, $p = 0.505$
The support I get from my work colleagues	3.90	3.90	3.78	3.70	$F = 1.39$, $p = 0.244$
The amount of responsibility I am given	3.52	3.55	3.71	3.57	$F = 1.24$, $p = 0.294$
The opportunities I have to use my skills	3.36	3.42	3.63	3.50	$F = 1.96$, $p = 0.119$
The extent to which the Trust values my work	2.99	2.84	2.73	2.96	$F = 1.83$, $p = 0.140$
My level of pay	2.36	2.41	2.27	2.42	$F = 0.52$, $p = 0.666$
SCALE: Job satisfaction	**3.36**	**3.29**	**3.35**	**3.28**	**$F = 0.40$, $p = 0.750$**

Table 7.8 Intention to leave (mean score)

	South	Midlands	North	London	p-value
I often think about leaving this Trust	2.28	2.22	2.68	2.43	$F = 4.51$, $p = 0.004$
I will probably look for a job at a new organization in the next 12 months	1.99	1.96	2.23	2.04	$F = 1.96$, $p = 0.119$
As soon as I can find another job, I will leave this Trust	1.84	1.85	2.13	2.01	$F = 2.70$, $p = 0.045$
SCALE: Intention to leave	**2.14**	**2.29**	**2.39**	**2.35**	**$F = 3.52$, $p = 0.015$**

Where HCA–doctor contact took place, it could be:

- Tense:

  Field note_Midlands: The observee spotted a doctor talking to a patient she had previously been speaking to. The observee noticed that the doctor was labouring in the conversation and went to clarify that what the patient wanted was an update about what would be happening to him test/procedure wise over the next couple of days. The doctor brusquely replied 'I *am* updating him', and it was evident from her demeanour that the observee felt embarrassed or belittled.

- Conflictual:

  HCA_Midlands: We had the sign out, barrier nursing in progress, please wear gloves and aprons before and after attending. So obviously this doctor thought this doesn't apply to him. So off he trots in to the bay with no gloves, no aprons on and we stopped the doctor and said 'look, you know, you need to come in, read the sign'. And then we got reported that we were being so rude.

- Patronizing—as reflected in doctors' views about HCAs:

  Doctor_Midlands: Some auxiliaries can be disruptive. I mean a lot of them don't come from a nice middle class background, they come from, you know a slightly different social sphere and they have different personalities and character to some of the nurses on the ward, and the doctors for that matter. Some, they have a different outlook on life and different mannerisms and characteristics and sometimes that becomes irritating and a nuisance.

  HCA_South: Sometimes some of them [doctors] look at us and they know that we're not qualified so they don't really listen to what we're saying, they don't take it onboard.

- Nasty:

  HCA_South: I have had a few [doctors] who have been particularly nasty, and I mean nasty, but having said that, there's been a few who have been absolutely wonderful as well. But when they've been nasty they've been really nasty ... Nasty in the sense of putting our roles down, and I think one doctor made a magnificent display, he called our jobs 'menial and meaningless' ... to my face, yes, in the staffroom. That was rather upsetting.

In the main, HCAs perceived relations with registered nurses in a positive light. Certainly, there was an acknowledged unevenness in such relations, some HCAs viewing the quality of interaction with nurses as contingent upon various factors. In the main, however, HCAs saw registered nurses as inclusive and supportive:

> HCA_London: On the whole they're [relations with nurses] very good. It just depends again which nurses are working with us and how much they're helping us. We can take it that they have their own jobs to do but what we don't like is if we are running around like lunatics and they're sitting at the desk doing paperwork that perhaps one of them can do or it could wait.
> HCA_North: Some of them [nurses] are hard work and some of them aren't but I mean you do spot that, don't you? But they're all nice and they've all got a sense of humour, which I was quite surprised because I've got a sense of humour and that's one thing I like. And especially the men, they've got a really good sense of humour. But they are, they're all really, really nice people, I can't ask for a better bunch.

At the same time there was evidence, hinted at in the earlier comments, of certain tensions. It is worth recounting at length an instance of HCA–nurse conflict, indicative of a residual and quite deep-seated 'them–us' mentality:

> HCA_London: The last incident of the ward meeting, I wasn't involved but one of the healthcare assistants mentioned something, and it all kind of backfired and there was two HCAs in the meeting and two staff nurses and it kind of was 'them' and 'us'. You know, 'You don't tell us this' and, 'We don't tell you that' and dah, dah, dah, dah. And the healthcare assistant in question who doesn't very often speak out anyway really said something on behalf of another HCA who wasn't there, which she says she's never going to speak out again because of the reaction that she got … It was something to do with, it was so silly, it was like the [ward name] next door borrowed, came and took some sugar from our stock and we said, 'Oh what are you taking our sugar for?', you know. And they said, 'Oh apparently we are taking your sugar now, we've been taking your sugar, we're on the same budget' or whatever it was, whatever was said. And the girl said, 'I didn't know that', and I said, 'I've never heard that', and even someone else said, 'Oh I've never heard that'. And in the meeting they said that they would like to know, the healthcare assistant said, 'We'd like to know, you know, about the sugar because nobody's told us', because we're all doing the sugar and wondering where it's all going'.

Indeed many of the HCA 'dislikes' were raised in the context of their relationship with nurses. The following emerged from the qualitative research with some regularity:

* Lack of recognition and respect:
  HCA_London: The thing I hate the most is we are not supported, not one little bit, we're not paid or respected for the work that we do, because what I do now is what a nurse did three years ago, four years ago, and everybody gave them respect for what they did and paid them for what they did. So now three, four, five years on that I'm doing exactly the same role, why am I in a Band 2 and getting no respect for it?

HCA_South: I don't think we're as respected as much but, you know, you quite often hear people go, 'Oh she's only an HCA' or, you know, 'Oh that's an HCA's job', and that's a little bit degrading sometimes.

- Being the 'dirty workers':
  HCA_South: Sometimes the bells might be going and you know that it's probably someone wanting a commode, but they [nurses] might just say, 'Well can you get it', and it's like, 'Well what's the matter with you, what are you doing?'. 'Well I'm doing my writing.' Well I'm on another patient in another team so, you know, it's not even my team so really shouldn't, you know, lots of nurses do that and it does get on the HCA's nerves.

- Being the 'workhorse' and 'dumped on':
  HCA_North: The only thing I hate doing and it's not really my role though, it's just something that gets dumped on me quite often, when patients go home and you've got to clean the whole bed space and stuff.
  HCA_London: The only downsides really is when you do get a trained member of staff who just think you are a, a dogsbody.

Other HCA 'dislikes', less related to registered nurses, were also raised:

- The behaviour of patients and relatives:
  HCA_London: The least thing I like are the relatives. They just bombard you and some of them are so aggressive and you really do try your best and, you know, it's not always good enough and you just think, sometimes you think why do I bother, you know.

- Intense work pressures:
  HCA_North: The only thing I don't like about the job is really when I come on they are short-staffed and then the ward is busy, that's the only time I don't really like the job. Because you're rushing and you don't have time to do stuff, you're just rushing and doing everything, that's the only time I don't like it, when we're short-staffed.

Emotion at work

The emotional experiences of HCAs emerged as one of the more potent means of assessing the consequences of the role for its post holders. It was an area of interest opened-up in a fairly tentative way in interviews with HCAs in the early case studies. However, it was pursued more systematically as it became clear that emotional responses were a rich source of evidence on impact of the role on post holders. The data collected on emotion remained qualitative, drawn mainly from the interviews and to a lesser extent from our observational work.

There is an extensive literature on emotion at work (Bolton, 2005), and particularly on emotional labour (Hochschild, 1983). Healthcare work is often seen as an emotional zone (Fineman, 1993), the site for the expression and management of varied and intense emotion (Theodosius, 2008). Indeed there has been a range of studies exploring emotions at work amongst registered nurses (Smith, 1992; McCreight, 2005). These studies have not been extended to HCAs, a striking omission given, as revealed by our research, the development of the HCA as the principle bedside presence. This section does not connect directly to the emotion work literature (for such a discussion see Kessler et al., 2011, 2012b), but the value of exploring this issue here, and the source of its potency, lies in the light it sheds on HCA feelings and the HCAs' sensitive handling of other stakeholder feelings (see also Chapter 9).

The HCA role emerges from our work as emotionally intense, both in terms of the need for HCAs to manage their own emotions and to deal with the feelings of others on the ward, in particular patients, their relatives, and friends. The consequences of this emotional intensity on the working life of the HCA, and indeed on their broader well-being, were, however, far from straightforward. An assumption that emotional intensity either degraded or enriched the HCAs' work experience was too simplistic, failing to account for the myriad ways in which HCAs engaged with emotionally-charged situations. The consequences of emotional engagement were found to be contingent upon the circumstances surrounding an episode or event, and mediated by the ways in which the HCA coped with the situation.

In interview, HCAs were asked whether they had become particularly attached to a patient, and to recount their experiences of an emotionally-charged situation such as dealing with a dying patient or with last offices (the cleaning and laying out of the body after death). Many of the views presented, therefore, related to death and dying. The views expressed left little doubt that working as an HCA could have a profound emotional impact. It is worth reproducing one such story to illustrate this point:

> HCA_North's Story: At the time I didn't think it was real. What happened was [nurse's name] had said to me 'Oh this lady's really unwell', and … she asked me if I minded sitting with her; because she didn't have any family with her or anything, and she said that she could possibly die and how do I feel, you know, if I feel uncomfortable about doing it then don't do it, but she thought it would be a good learning opportunity. So I went and sat with her because I didn't mind … and as I was stroking her hand she did die and it was like it weren't real really. And I helped clean her and, and then when they wrapped her up … in the sheet, the thing that got to me most was actually covering her face, you know, wrapping her head up. I kept looking because I kept thinking I could see her breathing, and I was thinking, 'Oh'. Anyway I finished that shift … at three o'clock and … I had an appointment to try on wedding dresses and my mum was meeting me in the shop. And I went in and I was fine, I didn't feel upset or anything, but then when I started talking about it and I told my mum, I just burst into tears. And I just explained to her that it was when I wrapped the lady's head up that that's, that's what really got me really. I don't know why.

The self-contained nature of this story highlights the 'roller coaster' nature of the emotions experienced by the HCA: there is a momentum which builds and eventually leads to tears. It reveals the range of feelings likely to be experienced: the calm of being with the dying patient, a sense of detachment during last offices giving way to distress on meeting with her mother.

It needs to be stressed that such experiences and engagement with death and dying were not frequent. During our observation, there were typically dying patients on a ward, but there were only two shifts where patients died (two in quick succession on one shift) and one shift where there was a cardiac arrest. Nonetheless, such events remained an ever-present possibility, and emotional engagement was not solely confined to such situations.

The emotional response to dealing with death and dying amongst HCAs was found to be heavily dependent on the circumstances and on individual coping strategies. A number of circumstances were highlighted as shaping the HCA emotional reaction to such a situation: the age of the patient, the patient's length of stay, the predictability of the death, connections with personal experience, and the level of support available within and beyond the Trust.

The age of the patient

Emotional intensity was heightened where the patient was young:

> HCA_South: A few years ago somebody who was relatively young, in their 40s died, I fortunately wasn't here for the incident but I helped lay him out and that was, shocking is probably too hard a word, because I didn't know him, but that was unusual and that was probably something else to deal with.

The patient length of stay of the ward

Naturally, the longer the stay, the more staff come know the patient, and the keener the feelings if and when that patient dies:

> HCA_Midlands: If they've been with you a long time and pass away or something, it can be quite sad … sometimes you can't help your feelings.

The predictability of the death

The more sudden the death, the greater the emotional impact:

> HCA_Midlands: I'd been in that morning and I'd said to her [the patient] 'Blimin' hell you look ever so well today' … And I was chatting to her, she was fine … then I just finished giving my last dinner out and the crash alarm went off … She was in the chair and she's just slumped and they tried to resuscitate her a couple of times. I mean she was a good age, she was ninety-four I think. And I felt awful because I sat there and thought I'd just been speaking to her literally just over an hour ago and she was fine … that was the last time that I properly had a cry.

The extent to which an episode connected with a personal experience

Where a death is connected to a HCA's personal experience, the emotional response is likely to be more intense:

> HCA_Midlands: It never gets any easier but you learn to cope with it different, and that's the only way I can put it. It's like after I came back to work after my daughter died, I mean she was twenty-three so I found that, well obviously really hard, and when I first came back to work I could not deal with a dead body.

The level and nature of support available on the ward

The support from other HCAs and ward colleagues could mitigate the effects of an emotionally-charged situation:

> HCA_Midlands: I ask [new HCAs] to come in with me [to last offices] … But there's one thing I always say to them: 'If any part of that time you don't want to do anything and if you think I can't do this, just tell me'; I let them go out, I'll get somebody else; because it's not a nice job and not everybody can handle it.

The impact of these emotionally intense episodes was mediated by a number of coping strategies: the same event could have very different consequences depending on how the HCA interpreted and sought to rationalize the situation. The following coping strategies were identified: continuation of care, talking with the deceased, familiarization, keeping an emotional distance and seeing the patients as being at 'peace'.

Continuation of care

A number of HCAs managed by viewing last offices as a continuation of care; the final act they could perform for the patient:

> HCA_London: If you've nursed that patient or if you've been involved in that patient's care, when it does come to the end it's quite a nice thing to do in some respects because you've done the final bit.

Talking to the deceased

HCAs sometimes continued talking to the deceased patient as if they could still hear them and were still present:

> HCA_London: I talk to them, I like to do my best for them and in my eyes it's the last thing I can do for them, so I want them to look and smell lovely. And all the way through I talk to them as if they're still with us. Some you get quite attached to and it can be quite heart-rending, but in my mind they're at peace now, they're out of pain. So sometimes it's the better thing, and you just say your goodbye and even when the porters come to get them, they're quite fussy – be gentle with them, don't bang their head, we're there to help all the time.

> Patient_Midlands: And then our [HCA] came ... she sings a lot because she goes to church and it was [the HCA] who went to him and got him prepared for when the relatives came ... you couldn't see nothing, you could just hear [HCA] laying this man out and singing ... she was lovely.

Familiarization

HCAs differed as to whether familiarity with death softened its emotional impact over time. Some felt 'you never got used it', others suggested that it became somewhat easier to control emotional response with experience:

> HCA_North: It's like obviously now and again, when I first heard that somebody had died I did get upset, but I thought well it's the way of life now, got to cope with it. So I've coped really well since. Because I think if I'd, if I had got attached, if I did get too close I wouldn't have been here, I'd of left by now, so. But you do get slightly close, but not too.

Keeping an emotional distance

Some HCAs dealt with situations by keeping their emotional distance. This was rationalized in slightly different ways: for some it was linked to 'professionalism'—an expected requirement of the job; for others it was more a matter of self-preservation—being continually drawn into situations would be too emotionally draining; for yet others direct engagement was seen as an intrusion into other peoples' concerns:

> HCA_London: I do tend to distance, I don't like to get too involved. Sometimes you can get a bit too involved and I don't think that's professional. Sometimes the girls do get a bit, you know, like they kiss and cuddle them and I sort of, it's just me I suppose, I'm just, I don't think you should do that. But yes, be polite to people and, you know, show compassion and all that, but I don't think you should get, well I don't know, I just don't think it's right, but that's me.

Patients at peace

Some HCAs managed by consoling themselves that the patient was at 'at peace' and no longer in pain:

> HCA_North: [On] odd occasions you still think about it depending on what situation that patient has died in. And if they've sort of gone to sleep or it's been a patient that is terminally ill, it's easier because they're not suffering anymore.

Summary

The consequences of the HCA role for post holders were conceptualized in positive and negative terms: the basis for a more fulfilling working life, well rewarded and providing greater career opportunities or a source of work intensification, poorly remunerated and with little scope for progression.

The findings presented in this chapter suggest that on balance the role was seen more in a positive than a negative light, particularly by those performing it. This is not to overlook the contradictory outcomes of the role for post holders, or evidence to suggest that these positive HCA views had emerged not because of the way they were treated but rather despite it.

In general HCAs enjoyed their job. They were especially keen on those aspects of their work which involved patient contact, and displayed aspirations to develop either within their current role or by moving into registered nursing. This positive outlook was confirmed by high levels of job satisfaction and a low intention to leave their Trust. These findings might be related to our discussion of HCA backgrounds: given the life and work experiences of many post holders, the HCA role represented an unusual and welcome opportunity to engage in what they felt was meaningful work and to develop themselves. Indeed, placing the role in this context helps explain the HCAs' positive views of the role despite findings which raised questions about how well they were managed, their sometimes tense relations with other team members and the barriers faced in realizing their ambitions.

The management of HCAs was revealed as uneven, both between Trusts and between policy areas. The variable treatment of HCAs by Trusts was particularly stark in relation to induction and NVQ accreditation and induction. In other policy areas, the management of HCAs was often weak across the Trusts: a dedicated HCA voice within Trusts was largely absent while the completion of performance appraisals was patchy. These concerns about the management of HCAs were at their most acute in relation to pay and grading. There was a (mis)alignment between pay, NVQ qualifications, and the actual tasks performed by post holders. Indeed, it was suggested that with the concentration of HCAs in Band 2, post holders were often over-qualified and or engaged in activities beyond what might normally be expected from those in this band, a situation which might be viewed as 'unfair'.

Relations with other team members, particularly registered nurses, were perceived as cordial and constructive, but there were some perceived tensions. There were concerns about a lack of respect and recognition, and about their role as the ward's 'work horse' and 'dirty worker'. In terms of aspiration, most HCAs were content to remain within their role, but also keen to develop within it. This is not to discount a significant minority of HCAs who retained nurse aspiration and saw their future in such a role. The scope for HCAs to advance these in-role and out-of-role ambitions in practice were, however, constrained. In part HCAs had to overcome personal barriers to their development: the limits on their time, energy and resources. At the same time, the support provided by Trusts to support the HCA in these terms was somewhat questionable.

As implied, the consequences of the HCA role for post holders were not readily classified as unambiguously positive or negative, often combining elements of both. This was most clearly reflected in the emotional engagement of HCAs with their work. As the main bedside presence, the emotions managed by HCAs—their own and those of others—were often intense. For the HCA such emotion management was stressful and the source of distress; at the same time the ability to provide comfort at the most difficult of times was commonly seen as the most rewarding part of the job.

Issues for reflection

The findings in this part of the report suggest the need for Trusts to consider the following in respect to consequences for HCAs:

- The greater use of induction to better prepare HCAs for different aspects of their role and to more effectively manage and shape their expectations about the role and their futures.

- The development of a more effective collective voice for HCAs.

- The consequences of a misalignment between pay band, NVQ qualifications, and tasks performed: for example, whether HCAs with NVQ 3 on pay Band 2 are withholding capabilities or underpaid for their delivery.

- The residual dissatisfactions with pay amongst HCAs.

- The lack of recognition and respect perceived by some HCAs.

- The comprehensive completion of PDRs for HCAs as a means of developing HCA futures in a more transparent, structured, and disciplined way.

- The emotional intensity of the HCA role and ways HCAs might be better supported in this respect.

Chapter 8

Consequences for nurses

Nurse_Midlands: They're a godsend basically, most of them, most of them.

Nurse_South: If you have a very good HCA, your shift is wonderful, if you have one that doesn't want to be there and doesn't actually do what they're meant to do properly and you're going behind them checking that they've washed the patients it makes life hard because you're not only doing your job but you're checking they've done theirs.

The development of the HCA role has been presented as creating a dilemma for registered nurses. It is a dilemma in part related to the nature of the nurse professionalization project. A project founded upon a deepening of technical skills amongst nurses, and a taking-on of more specialist tasks, would welcome the HCA role as a convenient depository for routine and 'burdensome' work. However, a project based on claims to the holistic provision of care by nurses, would look more critically on HCA encroachment into nursing, and view the delegation of tasks as problematic. In such circumstance it becomes pertinent to consider whether the HCA is viewed as advancing the nurse professionalization project or as hindering it.

A more prosaic, but overlapping, dilemma revolves around the balance nurses might seek between the support provided by the HCA to them and the additional supervisory responsibility implied by greater HCA involvement in the delivery of healthcare. It is a dilemma heightened by nurse accountability for the HCA which flows from such supervision, particularly within the context of nurse registration. The NMC Code of Practice is fairly clear on this issue, the registered nurse being responsible for the delegation of tasks to but not for their performance by the HCA. However, in practice the distinction between delegation and performance is not always clear cut, the lack of Trust guidance on this issue adding to the confusion.

Against the backdrop of these dilemmas, this chapter explores the impact of the HCA role on the registered nurse in three main ways: the first, whether and in what sense nurses value the HCA; the second, the circumstances in which the registered nurse might engage with the HCA, and the contingencies governing the nature and quality of this interaction with HCAs; and third, any tensions in this relationship, the form they take, whether and how they are resolved.

The chapter argues that, in general, and notwithstanding certain perceived difficulties in the relationship, nurses greatly value the contribution of HCAs to their working lives. A closer examination of the picture, however, suggests a slight disconnect between the qualitative and quantitative data on these issues: the former strongly endorses the significant, positive HCA contribution to the nurses' working lives, the latter provides a more qualified picture. The cause of this disconnect remains open to discussion. It might relate to the methodologies used, although given the plausibility of nurse ambiguities in the context of professionalization, it might also reflect a genuine uncertainty amongst nurses about how to view the HCA.

The value of the HCA: qualitative findings

The interview data suggested a strong consensus amongst nurses in all Trusts that HCAs added value to their working lives. The following statements from nurses are fairly typical, the general view being that HCAs were an essential part of the ward team and crucial in facilitating the performance of their role:

> Matron_South: Nurses for the most part have a huge amount of admiration for HCAs and … a good HCA is utterly invaluable; and an integral part of the team, without exception really. Trained nurses recognise that they couldn't do their job if they didn't have the support of the HCAs.
>
> Nurse_London: There are big positives to having them [HCAs] … We couldn't do our jobs without them being there to support us. They're a big asset for doing the things perhaps I would like to do, you know, but I've got other things that I have to do like the paperwork and things like that. Whereas they haven't got to worry about that and can go and do, just do the little things that make the patients' stay a bit more comfortable really.
>
> Nurse_North: If I ain't got a healthcare, it's a big impact; it makes my job so much harder. And it's only when you haven't got one you realise how much you appreciate them.
>
> Senior nurse_Midlands: I couldn't really manage the ward without them. I always say to them they're the backbone of the ward really. And I do say that to them because I don't think we could manage to function without them.

The HCA contribution to the nurse was explored in an opened-ended and grounded way in the interviews, with a question to nurses on how they viewed the HCA role. Such an approach prompted nurses to raise a variety of ways in which HCAs helped them, some overlapping with those raised by policymakers—a relief and a co-producer—but others more novel and precisely conceived. The following, often overlapping, contributions made by HCAs were highlighted by nurses: relief; partner; mentor; extra 'pair of eyes'; co-producer; and proxy. Each will be considered in turn.

Relief

Nurses most commonly cited the HCA's contribution as a relief. This involved the delegation by nurses of routine tasks to the HCA so allowing the nurse to concentrate on other priorities. In effect the HCA was left alone or with an HCA colleague to carry out work that the nurse might otherwise have performed, so freeing up the nurse for other activities:

> Nurse_London: We've got some really good HCAs, it makes me feel that I can concentrate on some of the things I do, it might be with the paperwork that you have to catch up, and I feel that I can concentrate on that a bit more without worrying about things not being done on the ward, without worrying about the obs not being done or something like that.
> Nurse_Midlands: They [HCAs] can make our job a lot easier because if we've got discharges they'll always make sure that the bed area's cleaned and ready for the next patient, so you can just get on with admitting the next beds. If they weren't there we'd have to go and do that as well.
> Nurse_South: They make it easier because they are there, you know that even if you're off doing phone calls or filling in forms or sorting out drugs, they are still there plodding through doing the care, coming and telling you if there's a problem, and just getting on with it.
> Ward manager_North: [HCAs] make [the nurses'] role somewhat easier because they've got time to free themselves to be doing other things like answering patient queries, looking, doing the post op care, getting patients ready for theatre, checklists and things.

Partner

If the use of the HCA as a relief involved the delegation of tasks, the nurses' use of the HCA as a partner was based upon the nurse and HCA working together, in, for example, making a bed or washing a patient:

> Nurse_North: When I need help like washing a patient, the other nurse, maybe we're only two nurses on the ward, the other nurse is busy, I will just ask the healthcare to help me.

Alternatively HCAs and nurses might work as partners in tandem on complementary activities. In the following case the nurse was dealing with the admission of a patient while the HCA took observations:

> Nurse_North: Like when we are doing admissions, when the patient arrive on the ward the first thing they do, they [HCAs] do the observations while I'm checking

what's wrong with the patient, and then when they give me the observations I look at them and then see if the patient needs a doctor just there and then.

Another example of complementary partnership working, a 'good cop, bad cop' routine, was picked up during research observations:

Field note_North (Medical): The Band 6 coordinator gruffly barked at a patient to get out of bed after which the observee [an HCA] was quick to come over and explain in a more gentle and persuasive manner.

Mentor

HCAs, particularly those with experience were sometimes the repository and guardians of ward practice and norms, and could be an important source of informal and formal knowledge and guidance not only to new HCAs but to student nurses and, indeed, newer registered nurses:

Nurse_London: It's actually good to have HCAs on the ward, they know a lot of things, loads of things. When I first started as a newly qualified they actually helped me a lot to go through my ten months here, because they've been there quite long and they know what they're doing. They are professional, they play a good role in the ward and they know what they're doing, and I'm very happy to have them around. They are very knowledgeable.

As noted during research observation:

Field note_North: At the nurses' station where the observee [an HCA] recounted how she helped comfort a patient earlier on in the shift by talking him down through his anxiety and tears by getting him to talk about his earlier years. My impression was that the observee was taking the opportunity to pass on experience to a young [student nurse].

As implied in this last instance, at times this mentoring role could slip over into a teaching role, where nurses were learning on-the-job from the HCA:

Matron_Midlands: A lot of the newly qualified nurses learn an awful lot from the experienced auxiliary nurses; because in some of the areas, I mean especially on the respiratory ward you get patients that come in and out and they get known by the staff, so if you're new to that ward you can rely on a bit of history sometimes to manage some of those people.

Extra 'pair of eyes'

HCAs were seen to have a value to nurses in providing another pair of eyes: this might take the form of keeping a watching brief on patients and/or spotting important changes in the patient's conditions which could then be reported back to the nurse. It might be viewed as a form of 'arm's length' partnership working, the HCA being able to oversee a patient's condition in the absence of the nurse, and communicate relevant information:

> Nurse_South: If you know that person [HCA] really well and you've worked with them a long time … and you know that they've got a feel for certain things and they can come back to you and say 'I've been to see Mrs so and so, I don't think they look as well today as they did yesterday, I just gave them a wash and they're not acting like they were yesterday'. And certain HCAs can pick up on certain things and they've done the job for a long time, and they make your life a lot easier.

One story is worth recounting at length: it illustrates the value of HCAs as an 'extra pair' of eyes, albeit for the doctor. It highlights an HCA's confidence in critically challenging a professional, and in so doing providing a crucial safety net for care:

> Matron_Midlands: Certainly doctors will spot the good ones [HCAs] and grab them if they need a hand. Some of them [HCAs] are fabulous and I'll give you an example: in A&E the other day an auxiliary had done an ECG on a patient, and had been in the department years, took the ECG to a doctor and said 'could you have a look at this', and they said 'oh yes, that's fine'. And she looked at it herself again and thought that's never fine, so went and found a more senior doctor and said 'I've just shown this to the SHO and he says it's fine, but I don't think it is'. And it wasn't. So they are worth their weight in gold sometimes because, you know, there's a potential there for a serious incident.

Co-producer

The public policy emphasis on the HCA's contribution as a co-producer has been highlighted, but it is worth distinguishing between the distinctive contribution made by the HCA both from the nurse and from the patient perspective. These overlap in important respects: what is useful to the nurse, is often useful, albeit possibly less directly, to the patient. However, it remains analytically important to explore the HCA-as-co-producer contribution as perceived by these different stakeholders. In the next chapter we consider the patient's view of the HCA as co-producer, whilst focusing on nurse perceptions in this chapter.

Certainly, the HCA was seen by nurses to add something distinctive to nursing, with this contribution taking different forms. Given their personal backgrounds, HCAs were sometimes better able to connect to patients than nurses, therefore providing a 'bridge' for the nurse to the patient. For example, it was noted during one of our ward observations that a nurse called upon an HCA with the same ethnic background as a patient to translate: the patient could not speak English. Indeed HCAs often appeared able to elicit useful information and responses from a patient, less accessible to the nurse:

> HCA_Midlands: When I've assisted with a wash with the nurse present as well, the patients, they do tend to talk about their problems more, especially if they've got some

kind of relationship going with the auxiliary in front of the nurse then, so the nurse can pick up on.

Proxy

There were instances where nurses viewed HCAs as a proxy for themselves: the nurse was tied up in other work, and was happy to let the HCA act in their place. It is a role which comes closest to the notion of the HCA-as-nurse-substitute:

> Senior nurse_South: Quite often if the nurses are busy, patients will talk to the care workers and they will come and say to us there's this problem, 'oh the nurses are too busy'. And if they're a good HCA they can also spot, if you're busy with something or the other, that a patient isn't well and they will come and get you straightaway and say deal with this patient, it doesn't look good and that.

The value of the HCA: quantitative findings

In our surveys we focused on three forms of support provided by HCAs to nurses as revealed in the interviews: the relief, the mentor, and the additional pair of eyes. The HCA role as co-producer is more fully dealt with in Chapter 9, looking at the patient–HCA relationship.

While nurses in interview were generally effusive about the HCA contribution in these terms, the survey results were somewhat more mixed. As can be seen from Table 8.1, there was moderate support for the HCA as a relief, albeit with some variation between the Trusts: for example, the nurses in North had a slightly more positive view of the HCA-as-relief than the nurses in London. There was much weaker support amongst nurses for the HCA-as-mentor, again with some difference of view between Trusts: nurses in South were much less likely to see the HCA as a mentor than those in North. The measure of the HCA as an additional 'pair of eyes' did not scale particularly well (alpha = 0.48), but the separate items suggested only mixed nurse support for the HCA in this capacity: moderately strong on the statement on the HCA as a 'pair of eyes'; much weaker on the HCA spotting something that might have been missed.

This discrepancy between qualitative and quantitative data suggests some ambiguity on the part of nurses towards HCAs. It is an ambiguity which comes into sharper relief in considering the contingent nature of the HCA–nurse relationship and some of the concerns raised by nurses about the HCA role.

A contingent relationship

The nature of the nurse relationship with HCAs is influenced by two sets of related factors (see Figure 8.1): the first set focuses on how the individual HCA

Table 8.1 Value of the HCA to nurses: relief, mentor, another pair of eyes (mean score)

	South	Midlands	North	London	p-value
HCA as relief:					
HCAs carrying out direct care tasks has made my life easier	3.75	3.75	3.89	3.63	$F = 1.54$, $p = 0.203$
It is easier for me to get essential paperwork done with a HCA on the ward	3.43	3.53	3.83	3.13	$F = 9.65$, $p < 0.001$
Being able to delegate to a HCA makes a positive difference to my workload	4.01	3.92	4.07	3.93	$F = 1.23$, $p = 0.299$
SCALE: HCA as relief	**3.73**	**3.74**	**3.94**	**3.57**	**$F = 5.34$, $p = 0.001$**
HCA as mentor:					
HCAs will often be the first to show student nurses how to do things on the ward	2.14	2.81	3.00	2.79	$F = 19.27$, $p < .001$
Newly qualified nurses will often look to HCAs for advice	2.63	2.97	3.19	2.94	$F = 8.60$, $p < .001$
HCAs often help newly qualified nurses 'find their feet' on the ward	3.19	3.26	3.40	3.30	$F = 1.32$, $p = 0.268$
SCALE: HCA as mentor	**2.66**	**3.01**	**3.20**	**3.01**	**$F = 14.17$, $p < 0.001$**
HCA as another pair of eyes:					
I can rely on HCAs to let me know when there is something wrong with a patient	3.29	3.63	3.77	3.40	$F = 7.33$, $p < 0.001$
I regard HCAs as another pair of eyes on the ward	3.89	3.84	3.98	3.91	$F = 0.50$, $p = 0.680$
A HCA will sometimes spot something that I have missed	3.23	2.82	3.05	3.12	$F = 6.03$, $p < 0.001$
SCALE: HCA as another pair of eyes	**3.47**	**3.42**	**3.60**	**3.47**	**$F = 1.59$, $p = 0.191$**

is perceived by the nurse; and the second is connected to nurse characteristics which might shape how the nurse perceives the HCA.

Nurse views on the HCA

The nurse is unlikely to have a standard relationship with HCAs as a group of workers: a more personal, bespoke relationship more typically develops with

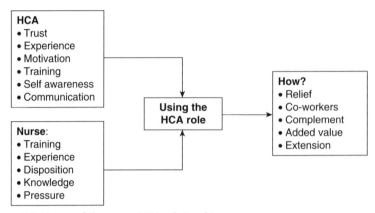

Figure 8.1 Nature of the nurse–HCA relationship.

different HCAs on the ward team. This relationship is rooted in the perceived characteristics, capabilities and attitudes of the HCAs. As Figure 8.1 indicates *the trust* held by the nurse in the HCA is crucial to how frequently they are used and for what purposes: the higher the trust the more frequent the nurse use of HCA and for more complex tasks:

> Senior nurse_South: It's difficult, you've got to have a lot of trust in the person you're delegating the job to; to know that they are (a) competent to do the job, (b) willing and (c) able to say I've done this job and tell you any differences that they might think. Whereas you might have someone else that will just come and do a blood pressure, write it down and walk off and not tell you, you've got to, it's kind of difficult but a lot of the healthcare assistants we've had a long time and they know the job just as good as we do and we depend on them really.

The importance of trust was highlighted by the difficulties nurses faced when bank and agency HCAs, with limited knowledge of the ward, its routines, and patients, came onto their shift:

> Nurse_North: We have a lot of issues with bank staff, both qualified and healthcare assistants, that seem to just come, do what they need to do, don't pass any information on, and you do sometimes feel that you're basically on your own and it sounds awful but you'd probably have been better without them there because you know what you're doing then and you're not having to go over and check their work over and over again; you should have just maybe done it yourself the first time, which is sad really.

It takes a while for a nurse to develop trust in an HCA, to be fully confident that tasks can be delegated to them. Such trust is often built on the nurse's *own experience* of working with the HCA:

> Nurse_North: [Trust] comes with experience with working alongside some of the HCAs. It's very difficult for you to trust a new healthcare assistant and you do

constantly sort of check their work for a short time until you feel that they're comfortable with what they're doing and that they know, you know, when they need to be telling you that something's wrong.

Nurse_London: It comes with years of experience because you can know the ones that are experienced from the ones [HCAs] who are not experienced, depending on what they do. Because as I say, when you do things you don't just take it for granted that it's done, you go and look at it. For example, as I said, if they go and empty the catheters, you see how they document what they emptied, you see what they document on the chart, how much the patient had to drink and whatever. So if over a period of time you're working with them and you're happy with what they're doing, then you develop confidence. But some, you have to be telling them always to do it, then you always have to be, you know, say 'oh I might as well do it myself' because I don't think she is sure what she's doing. So that's the difference. So just observing how they work.

It is this experience of working with an HCA that allows the nurse to develop a feel for the HCA's *capabilities,* facilitating an appreciation of what can safely be handed on. Where the registered nurse is assured, there are instances of a tacit acceptance that the HCA can perform tasks without continual reference to the nurse:

Ward manager_North: The qualified nurse should be delegating and guiding the clinical support worker throughout the shift. But because our support workers are so competent, they don't actually often need that. And like [two HCA names] they're both extremely competent and intelligent, and [HCA name] certainly should be a qualified nurse. But they know that they aren't qualified and they know that they mustn't just wade in and do a, a dressing … And the new ones don't because they don't have that experience … so if [two HCA names] are on I just think 'oh we're going to have a lovely day today', because I know that they will do everything that's expected of them and more … whereas the new ones are still being trained up.

This willingness to allow some HCAs a degree of free rein was also heavily dependent upon the nurse being comfortable with the HCA's *self-awareness*: there were task boundaries that the HCA should not cross, and the nurse needed to be sure that the HCA understood these boundaries, realized when they were being approached, and would not violate them. Some examples highlight the importance attached by nurses to the HCA's self-awareness:

Senior nurse_South: One of our healthcare assistants is fond of saying, 'you need to speak to a grown up' or 'I'll get my grown up' because she absolutely knows her limits and she's very experienced but she knows that she's the healthcare assistant and really doctors or the relatives need to be speaking to us.

Nurse_London: I'm worried that in some areas where maybe a healthcare assistant undertakes a series of clinical observations – temperature, pulse, respiration, blood pressure – that person's ability to recognise that there's something not quite right. And I think it's the wrong interpretation of observations and escalating, and recognising that there is a need to escalate that right now to the registered nurse.

The value placed on the HCAs' self awareness sits alongside the nurses' concern that the HCA can effectively communicate: the HCAs need to clearly articulate relevant information on say the patients' condition and the procedures they have completed. This is highlighted by one nurse from South:

> Nurse_South: If they can do all these things for you that's great, but if they can't communicate what they've done to you then you're in danger of sort of not actually knowing what's going on with your patients and missing vital signs, like if they took someone's obs and they had a pulse of forty, for example, and they didn't tell you then I would have a brachycardic patient about to arrest sitting there and I wouldn't know anything about it. So they need to make, you know, they can do these extra things but they need to be able to know how to use the results that they get from them.

Nurses pick up on the *disposition,* and particularly the *motivation,* of the HCA. Nurses are sensitive to different dimensions of the HCA's disposition. There is a lazy–active dimension: the more active the HCA, the more likely the nurse is to use them, while nurses display some care in keeping a watching brief on the less enthusiastic HCAs. This is highlighted by the following nurses:

> Nurse_South: We have one in particular [HCA] who doesn't like to work, you know, and you think 'oh gosh, I'm spending half my time chasing them around'. And she has been known to say 'I'm hiding from …' But she knows what I say, and I say 'I love you dearly but you're a nightmare'.
> Nurse_North: We've got another healthcare who you just can't trust quite so much. She's a bit lazy … she's more interested in going out for a cigarette every ten minutes and, I know and it's you can't trust her. She'll go off shift, and if she's been on a night shift she'd go off shift and like she should empty the catheters on a morning ready for the daytime, the catchers are not emptied.

There is also a proactive–reactive dimension, with the nurse displaying some preference for HCAs who are prepared to use their initiative, rather than waiting to be directed:

> Ward manager_North: There's one of the clinical support workers who's quite new; she will do anything that you ask her to do but if you don't ask her she just stands there. And we're working on that. And she'll stock up and she'll clean, because we have a weekly cleaning rota, she'll do everything but sometimes she'll just stand, and I can't stand it when people stand there and do nothing.
> Ward manager_North: The ones [HCAs] I find are the ones that take the initiative, they know what their role is and they're there to help with the washes and whatever else, and they get on and do the washes that they can do whilst you're doing pills.

Nurse characteristics

The second set of contingent factors influencing nurse views on, and engagement with, HCAs was associated with characteristics of the nurses themselves. This association needs to be treated with some care to avoid overgeneralizing, but Figure 8.1 suggests a number of influential features which emerged in the interviews. The age and experience of the nurse was mentioned with some regularity, younger or less experienced nurses tending either to underuse or overuse HCAs. It was a view held by HCAs, and to some extent confirmed by nurses:

HCA_South: It's the younger, the newer nurses coming in saying, they obviously don't know me as well, 'oh can you do this' or 'can't you do it?', what can you do, you know. So I think it's the older generation that allow me to do what I can do.

Matron_Midlands: Certainly the more experienced nurses would understand their [HCAs'] value. It's the newly qualifieds, suddenly they're, the qualified nurse, I'm the big I am, I've got me stripes on me shoulder now, and they forget their place sometimes I think.

Senior nurse_South: There are some [nurses] that perhaps don't trust them [HCAs] enough perhaps, particularly with new nurses that come on. Our healthcares are good in the fact they do a lot on this ward, I mean more than a lot of wards, they can do admissions, and I think some nurses are quite surprised at first but they realise that yes, they can do it and they're very competent, they're doing a lot of tasks.

Ward manager_Midlands: It's just, probably the junior nurse I think sometimes because they probably struggle with their workload less because they're newly qualified, suddenly they've got everything to do, and it's like, they're fighting between their documentation and keeping up with their cardex and, the obs and somebody's buzzing in another bay. So they probably don't appreciate them but rely on them [HCAs] more.

Just as the HCA's disposition affected how the nurse viewed and used them, so the nurse's disposition could influence how they regarded HCAs. There were some nurses who were simply 'lazy', consequently drawing heavily upon the HCAs.

Senior nurse_South: This is going to sound really bad but you know the nurses that are particularly, are lazy, for want of another word, they don't want to sit there and have to do this, this and this to patients, they'd quite happily sit on a chair and let the HCA do it and then do all the writing afterwards. Which is not really of any use to anyone, but there's people like that.

Others were very fixed in their views about the role of the HCA, and the tasks they should be performing:

Senior nurse_Midlands: Some nurses depend on a lot from an auxiliary, think the auxiliary should automatically do everything, like TEDS and stuff and beds and stuff, they don't want to do that job. Whereas some nurses will just think I better do it, I'll just get on with it and do it, and I think that's where you're, you can find you get the tension because they'll say 'oh bloody hell, I'm working with her again, she's going to make me do all the work'. And some auxiliaries won't, can't say no or find it difficult to, to stick up to some of the people. And so that's where you probably get the most tension.

These opinions were not solely linked to personality but might also be related to personal experiences or training:

> Senior nurse_North: Where you've been trained or where you've worked before determines how, how you treat your healthcare assistants. I worked on a ward very similar to this where you used them as much as you could get out of them and you really pushed them to do as much as they could. Sometimes you see nurses just expecting that they should just get everybody up and everybody washed and that's just their job and leave everything, leave all the bloods to me, I'll do it, instead of really pushing and developing people.

The cultural background of nurses was also alluded to by some as influencing nurse disposition towards HCAs:

> Nurse_North: Some of the HCAs are a bit strong, you find that like the Pilipino nurses are pretty quiet and they won't speak out for themselves. So rather than just sort of confront them they'll just do the obs themselves rather than saying come on, this is your, you do it, help me with this, they'll just get on with it and do it themselves like because they just don't like that confrontation with them. And I think sometimes that the HCAs can take advantage of the Pilipino nurses.
>
> Sister_South: Sometimes some of the overseas nurses might expect more from the support workers and that might be because of what they're used to, where they trained or where they worked before. But it doesn't last for long, and I think when they see how things are done and again if somebody comes to me and says they're being asked to do ridiculous things or being asked to do everything by a particular nurse, then I would speak to them and, you know, just point out how things are done.
>
> Sister_South: If you get, especially Spanish nurses because traditionally they don't wash patients, they don't give commodes to patients. That could cause friction because they could be sitting there doing nothing and the HCA's running around and running around and running around, and they'll say 'oh can you give us a hand', and they're like 'no, that's not my role'.

Tensions

The qualitative data suggested that from a nurse perspective the relationship with HCAs was not generally problematic. When asked whether there were any tensions with HCAs, a simple 'no' was not an uncommon response from a nurse. If probed further, examples given generally related to personality clashes rather than to any generic feature associated with HCAs as a group. However, some tensions were raised and observed. They included the following: 'them and us', misconceptions, accountability, and role boundaries.

Them and us

The divide between nurses and HCAs on some wards should not be overlooked. It has been noted that there were important differences in the backgrounds of nurses and HCAs, as well as in the tasks performed. In some cases this gave rise to a 'them and us' divide. This 'them' and 'us' mentality has been noted from an HCA perspective, and found an echo in the views of some nurses:

> Nurse_North: I don't really like ward meetings, it just turns into a big bitch fest. It does. But this one, we had a ward meeting and by the end of it I felt like slitting my wrists, I'm like what do I do that's any good ever, do you know? They [the HCAs] had a list! And a staff nurse asked a healthcare to do a blood sugar and the staff nurse heard her go, 'Well that could go on the list as well'. 'Well, if you don't want to do the obs, you don't do blood sugars, why should you do all the washes? Well what the hell else can you do on the ward?' Do you know what I mean? 'Well what do you want to do? Do you want to sit down and I'll bring you a cup of tea? Because that's not going to work'. It is very much them and us. It's shocking.
>
> Nurse_North: If [HCAs are] all on together then they'll all go for break together, and then like the staff nurses, obviously we all can't go for a break together, so like we don't go to break until half eleven and then you've got to have your dinner and it just screws your time. If they're not on together as friends, I mean they should work together as friends, but in the sense of they want to go to break together, they'll chat together, they'll talk in sluice together, and then you'll lose them for an hour.

Misconceptions

Nurses were sometimes resentful about how HCAs perceived the nurse role. In not always being engaged intensely in direct and indirect care, nurses were aware that HCAs sometimes viewed them as 'lazing about'. This could cause frustration amongst nurses who saw this as an HCA failure to appreciate the responsibilities and pressures they faced:

> Nurse_North: People like talk and talk and talk, like they know there's a lot of negativity between the healthcares, they feel like they're, well skivvies really, that's the term they've been using and like they're making all the beds, they're seen as being like beneath everybody else and they're made to do all the work. But I don't think they specifically understand what we've [nurses] got to do. I mean they've got observations, they've got to wash people and observations, but we've got the medications, admissions, discharge, there's things they can't do which we need to do.
>
> Nurse_London: I can remember being on a ward as a healthcare assistant and thinking the nurses ain't doing anything, they've been sitting down all morning, I've done all the washes, I've done this, I've done that. But now, having qualified and been a nurse, I can see the other side that actually yes, they may be sitting down at the desk but they're doing the admission, they're doing the discharge, you know, they're speaking to relatives. And sometimes I think the healthcare assistant forgets that but I also think the nurse forgets what actually they are asking them to do.

Accountability

The most tangible source of nurse tension related to the issue of accountability: both the HCAs' accountability for their work and how this affected nurse accountability. The former was reflected in nurse concerns about the ability of HCAs to understand and interpret the consequences of their actions: it was one thing to undertake an observation; another to interpret the reading and know that there was a problem. This broadened into a deeper worry about the absence of any national regulation of HCA activities. This concern was seen to overlap with worries about the nurses' own accountability for HCAs. In the absence of HCA registration, nurses were denied a form of quality assurance over the capability of the HCA. Attention has already been drawn to the importance of trust in these circumstances, and the time it might take for a nurse to build some confidence in HCA capabilities: there were residual concerns that ultimately it was the nurse registration that was 'on the line':

> Nurse_London: They [HCAs] need some sort of regulatory body or something because at the moment they're doing bloods or they do a plaster. As a registered nurse we are overall accountable for that. And even though they've gone through the course and everything we have to constantly monitor them because it's our registration on the line. I just think that if there was some sort of regulatory body that would strengthen their profession, they could use all these skills that they've been trained to do but can't use in practice, and they'd be able to use them in practice and they'd be accountable. And I think, yes, as a nurse, I think that would increase the standards.

While nurses generally appreciated the formal limits of their accountability as set out in the NMC guidance, with responsibility for the delegation of the activities but not their performance, there were complications in this relationship. For example, as already implied, weaknesses in Trust guidance left some doubt in the nurses' mind as to what could legitimately be delegated to the HCA:

> Manager_London: I think they're [nurses] jumpy because they're unsure on what they will be held accountable for. It works different with different nurses as well. There's some staff nurses out there that are quite happy for the HCAs to go off and do all these things. There's others go, 'Hold on a minute, you know, I'm accountable for that'.

Indeed, there were instances where ward managers stressed this nurse responsibility for the HCA:

> Ward manager_North: I try and make it clear to the qualified nurse that actually they are responsible and not the clinical support worker, and they need to be checking that everything's done because they're, they are given a lot of responsibility on here. I would say if anything more say than they should be.

Arguably this blunt ward manager's message to nurses, exacerbated nurse concerns when the more nuanced NMC guidance might have been more appropriate. However, the line between responsibility for delegation and responsibility for the task itself could be a thin one: if an HCA performed poorly should the nurse have been aware of this possibility before delegating? Rightly or wrongly, there was a degree of sensitivity to this issue and a sense of vulnerability amongst some nurses.

While important, these concerns should not be overstated. Our survey developed a three-item scale on whether nurses viewed HCAs as a 'burden', asking direct questions on whether nurses were worried about delegating to HCAs and about HCA understanding of what they were doing. As Table 8.2 notes, there are some significant differences between Trusts, with nurses in London significantly more likely to view the HCA as a 'burden'. However, in all four Trusts the means scores are low, well below the mid-point of our five-point scale, suggesting only weak support for this view.

Role boundaries

Tensions over role boundaries might be envisaged at different ends of a spectrum of nurse activities. At the more complex and technical extreme, HCAs performing an extended role might be seen as encroaching on core nurse activities. At the other, direct patient care extreme, HCA dominance might be seen to challenge nurse claims to the provision of holistic care (see earlier section). The qualitative fieldwork revealed little nurse concern about HCA activities at either end of the spectrum, although the occasional story was told which illustrated strains at the boundaries of the two roles. This is highlighted

Table 8.2 HCA as a burden (mean score)

	South	Midlands	North	London	p-value
Managing a HCA on a shift is a burden	1.94	1.88	1.55	2.15	$F = 7.78$, $p < 0.001$
Being accountable for the delegation of tasks to HCAs is a constant worry for me	2.41	2.39	2.25	2.57	$F = 2.28$, $p = 0.079$
I am always confident that HCAs fully understand what they are doing on the ward[a]	3.36	3.35	3.53	3.42	$F = 0.96$, $p = 0.412$
SCALE: HCA as a burden	**2.33**	**2.30**	**2.09**	**2.44**	**$F = 5.02$**, **$p = 0.002$**

[a] Scoring reversed when item included in the scale

by a matron in North voicing some general concerns about boundaries given the relative levels of training received by nurses and HCAs:

> Matron_North: There's responsibility, and accountability ... we've received a lot of training to do what we do and then if you look at the training of the healthcare support workers ... So I think there needs to be clear boundaries about what they can and can't do, and that's why I think it needs to be the basic nursing care and things.

At the more technical end, an HCA recounts an episode related to female catheterization where, slipping across a boundary, the limits of the HCA role were firmly imposed:

> HCA_London: So we took the decision to re-catheterise her because the trained nurse we wanted to talk to was in a meeting. Well we actually got carpeted for that, but afterwards when we did our rationale and said look, the reason was we didn't feel the bladder wash out was good enough, it didn't go in, to me it had only gone up the tube [10 ml], it had got no further, this lady was going to have a problem, and surely it's our responsibility to make sure she was OK for going home. So on that aspect we overstepped the mark because we needed to have a trained nurse's OK, but in our defence, our patient needed that doing.

At the other end, some concerns at the flight of nurses from direct care were raised:

> Manager_London: Our healthcare assistants do a lot of the hands-on care. It sort of goes against the grain for me because I was trained when actually the nurses, we did all the hands-on care as well. And I don't like this idea, healthcare assistants, don't get me wrong, they absolutely have their place, they're really valuable members of the team, but I don't like to see trained nurses completely standing back and not getting involved in hands-on care which I think potentially sometimes can happen.

Equally noteworthy were the findings from our surveys which explored role tensions. As a means of establishing such tension, nurses and HCAs were given a list of statements on who was most likely to perform certain routine, perhaps 'burdensome and 'dirty', direct and indirect healthcare tasks. As Table 8.3 indicates, a clear pattern emerges across all Trusts suggesting different nurse and HCA views on who engages with these activities: while nurses continue to see themselves as carrying out many direct and indirect care tasks, HCAs in contrast regard it as more likely that they carry out these activities. For example, it can be seen that there is moderate support amongst nurses for the suggestion that they will answer a buzzer before an HCA and usually empty a patient's commode. However, there is little support from HCAs for these assertions, implying rather that it is they who typically do this type of work. These are findings which suggest that nurses and HCAs have very different conceptions about their respective roles when it comes to the delivery of direct

Table 8.3 Role tensions (mean score)

	South		Midlands		North		London		p-value	
	HCAs	Nurses	HCAs	Nurses	HCAs	Nurses	HCAs	Nurses	HCAs	Nurses
A nurse will usually answer a patient's buzzer before a HCA[a]	1.84	3.13	1.99	3.08	1.94	2.96	1.79	3.23	$F = 1.26$, $p = 0.288$	$F = 1.69$, $p = 0.168$
It is usually a nurse that will empty a patient's commode[a]	1.83	3.35	1.95	3.13	1.94	3.13	1.68	3.46	$F = 2.28$, $p = 0.078$	$F = 3.78$, $p = 0.010$
Nurses rely on HCAs to do all the 'heavy' work	3.54	1.80	3.70	1.81	3.36	1.85	3.78	1.78	$F = 2.97$, $p = 0.031$	$F = 1.83$, $p = 0.908$
SCALE: Role tensions[b]	**3.96**	**2.44**	**3.92**	**2.53**	**3.82**	**2.59**	**4.09**	**2.35**	**$F = 2.55$, $p = 0.055$**	**$F = 3.02$, $p = 0.029$**

[a] Scoring reversed when item included in the scale, thus scale mean reflects 'tension' from the HCA point of view

[b] Two-way ANOVA main effects: Role, $F = 1194.07$, $p < 0.001$; Trust, $F = 0.11$, $p = 0.955$

and indirect patient care: while nurses continue to hold the view that they remain heavily involved in such activities, HCAs, for 'better or worse' see this as their territory. It is a difference of perception which might be seen to underlie some of the latent tensions in the nurse–HCA relationship: if the respective groups feel that they rather than the other perform these routine and onerous tasks, it is perhaps unsurprising that resentments occasionally creep into relations.

Summary

The HCA role was presented as one that might constitute a 'mixed blessing' for registered nurses. It was a role with the potential to provide considerable support for the nurse. Indeed, it has been stressed that one of the key public policy objectives underpinning the promotion of the HCA role was to relieve nurses of certain routine and 'burdensome' tasks, allowing them in turn to concentrate on core professional activities. However, it was also suggested that HCAs presented various threats to registered nurses, and to their profession. At a fairly prosaic level, the HCA might represent an additional, perhaps unwanted, managerial and supervisory responsibility. The concerns around such a responsibility might assume a somewhat sharper form where the issue of nurse accountability for HCA work arose. At an even more fundamental level, the development of the HCA role might be seen to challenge the nurse professionalization project: most obviously where the HCA acted as a substitute for the nurse, so encroaching on traditional, and core registered nurse activities; more insidiously where HCAs became the main bedside presence so challenging the nurses' claim to be the holistic provider of care.

The findings presented in this chapter suggest that, in the main, nurses viewed HCAs in an extremely positive light: the predominant message to emerge was one of the HCA as a welcome and valued form of support. In a highly intense and pressured working environment, nurses were rarely too 'precious' to deny the value of the help provided to them by the HCA. In particular, the qualitative data highlighted HCA contributions to the working lives of nurses that went beyond a relief role: HCAs were seen a partner, an extra 'pair of eyes', a co-producer, a mentor, and a proxy. In short, HCAs were typically seen by nurses as an essential and 'treasured' member of the ward team.

This picture needs, however, to be qualified in three important respects. First, there was a slight mismatch between the qualitative and quantitative data on nurse views of HCAs. This should not be overstated: thus the nurse surveys revealed that across all Trusts there was very little support for the view that

HCAs were seen by nurses as a 'burden' on them. However, these surveys did reveal a more grudging acknowledgement of the HCA contribution as a mentor and, to a lesser extent, as another 'pair of eyes', than revealed in our interviews with nurses. More striking were the very different conceptions held by nurses and HCAs of their respective contributions to the performance of certain routine, dirty, and onerous tasks. While stressing in interview the role of the HCA in relieving them of such tasks, in the survey nurses still felt that they were the ones performing such tasks, at the same time as HCAs saw themselves undertaking them.

This disconnect between the qualitative and quantitative material might lie in the relationship between methodologies and the kind of data generated. It is interesting to speculate on whether face-to-face interviews were more likely to encourage the nurse to present positive views on the HCA, than the more impersonal and private completion of a survey questionnaire. However, given the plausibility of nurse ambiguities towards the HCA, the contradictory evidence might well be seen to have picked up a genuine uncertainty amongst registered nurses as to how to view and treat workers in this role.

The second qualification to the picture presented relates to the contingent nature of nurse views on and engagement with the HCA. A range of factors were identified as affecting how nurses regarded and treated HCAs. The most significant was the level of nurse trust in the HCA: such trust took a considerable time to develop, and indeed its absence, highlighted where bank or agency HCAs were used, placed a considerable responsibility on nurses to ensure that tasks were satisfactorily performed. Nurse relations with HCAs were also seen as dependent on the perceived capabilities and motivation of the HCA. It was suggested that the nurse perspective on HCAs was not idiosyncratic to the individual nurse but might well be related to the age and experience of the nurse, as well as to their ethnic backgrounds.

The third qualification is associated with the residual tensions that nurses still perceived in their relations with HCAs. The most noteworthy of these tensions revolved around nurse accountability for HCAs. This was more than a concern about added managerial responsibility for the HCA, shading into a more profound worry about registration if a nurse failed to supervise an HCA appropriately. It was a worry exacerbated by the absence of Trust guidance on this issue and by the blunt advice sometimes given by ward managers: indeed the information provided to nurses on accountability might be seen to encourage nurse misconception of their responsibilities for the HCA. Whether well founded or not, these nurse fears were genuine enough, and indeed might be viewed as reflecting a real uncertainty about where responsibility lay in the 'hurly burly' of care delivery.

Issues for reflection

The findings in this part of the report suggest the need for Trusts to consider the following in respect to consequences of the HCA role for nurses:

• Fostering a greater mutual recognition between nurses and HCAs on their respective contributions of the patient care and functioning of the ward.

• Greater clarity on the tasks which might legitimately be delegated to HCAs so reducing nurse concern about their accountability for HCA performance.

• Some ongoing sensitivity amongst nurses about role boundaries.

Chapter 9

Consequences for patients

Nurse_Midlands: They [HCAs] can appear a little bit closer to the patient; they can get a bit more of a rapport.

Ward manager_South: If the patient thinks they're [an HCA] not a trained nurse they'll say 'well you're not a trained nurse, I don't want you'.

Introduction

The consequences of the HCA role for the hospital patient might be seen as 'the bottom line' issue for this study: after all, for policymakers and practitioners at national and Trust level, the main purpose of developing the HCA role might be viewed as the improvement of healthcare quality and the patient experience. The consequences of the HCA role for post holders themselves and for registered nurses might impact on patients in various, albeit indirect, ways: for example, how HCAs feel about their role is likely to impact on how enthusiastically they engage with patients; while nurse views on and management of HCAs as part of the ward team are also likely to affect the patient journey. In this chapter, however, we focus on the more direct impact of the HCA role on patients.

It will be recalled that the consequences of the HCA role for the patient were presented as assuming three possible forms. The first emerges as a positive scenario: the patient engages with the HCA as a more accessible source of care. In this case the HCA is regarded as a less intimidating, more approachable route to care than perhaps the nurse or other care professionals. Such outcomes derive from the greater availability of the HCA at the bedside, but also from the nature of the HCA role and from those who fill it: as a 'low-level' role the HCA might appear to the patient as less daunting, while in terms of personal background, patients might find more in common with the HCA than the nurse and consequently find it easier to relate to them.

The second possibility arises as a more negative scenario: the patient views engagement with the HCA as compromising care quality. As an unregulated role, the patient might well view treatment by the HCA as 'second best' to that received from the nurse professional, and lacking the necessary guarantees on competence and safety. Once more, a third scenario presents itself, with the HCAs' impact on the patient somewhat contradictory, with elements of the first and second scenarios combining themselves in a fluid and perhaps unstable way.

In unpacking these three possibilities and establishing their evidence base, the following issues were considered:

• Whether patients could distinguish between HCAs and nurses: how patients viewed and engaged with the HCA might well be related to whether they could tell the difference between different members of the nursing team.

• Whether patients had a distinctive relationship with HCAs: regardless of whether patients could distinguish HCAs from nurses, they might still, less knowingly, have developed a different relationship with them.

• Whether the identification and nature of the relationship with the HCA mattered in outcome terms: for example, whether patients felt more or less comfortable in dealing with HCAs than nurses on certain issues.

Our consideration of these issues was founded upon a rich data set: qualitative interview and observational data were available on HCA and nurse interaction with patients, while nurse and HCA survey material shed light on the relative incidence of caring behaviours and capabilities amongst these two occupational groups. Moreover, qualitative and quantitative data from the patients themselves, respectively from focus groups and surveys, provided a strong user perspective on how they viewed and engaged with HCAs. It was a wealth of data which not only brought the full range of stakeholder perspectives to bear on the HCA–patient relationship, but also provided an opportunity to explore whether the findings from these different sources were reinforcing or in tension with one another.

Unsurprisingly given these diverse data sources, the picture to emerge was complex, although a clear and coherent underlying story emerged. The complexity in part related to some disconnect between the data sources. There was quite a strong consensus from the HCA, nurse, and patient qualitative data that patients had a much closer and more open relationship with HCAs than nurses. The quantitative data collected, particularly, from nurses and patients, presented a much less clear cut picture, and hinted at some patient concerns with HCAs. The clear story to emerge, however, was that in all Trusts where patients could distinguish HCAs they had a markedly better care experience.

Distinguishing HCAs

A patient's ability to distinguish between HCAs and nurses might be expected to influence relationships between these different sets of actors: depending on how patients viewed the HCA, such recognition might encourage very different forms of interaction. In general, views from nurses and HCAs on the ability of patients to distinguish HCAs from other members of the ward team fell into a number of categories. First, there were those who felt that patients fairly readily distinguished HCAs:

> Matron_Midlands: Most people will work out straightaway, just by nature of what those professionals are coming and doing to them. So if it's the auxiliary nurse that's helping you to go to the toilet, then if you need a bedpan you'll tend to ask them. If it's the trained nurse who's giving you your painkillers, then when you want a tablet you'll ask them.

Second, there were some who questioned the capacity of patients to make a distinction between members of the nursing team:

> Nurse_London: I don't think a lot of patients know what a healthcare assistant is. We're constantly asked about the difference in uniform. I get called a doctor all the time, so I'm not sure if any patients know. But I think it's the uniforms as well, they're saying well what do the, the uniforms mean, what colour's a doctor, what colour's a nurse and you explain to them. But, you know, with a healthcare assistant, they view them as, as nurses, most of them anyway.

While third, there were a few respondents who felt that patients were not really concerned about being able to tell the difference:

> Ward manager_London: I suppose it depends what's being done to them, doesn't it? I mean some people would like to know it, wouldn't they, some can't be bothered I suppose, as long as they're being looked after and, you know, respectfully and properly.

Clearly Trusts sought to distinguish HCAs and other categories of staff in a number of ways. However, the effectiveness of these devices was often open to debate, providing some support for those who questioned the ability of patients to accurately tell the difference between staff members, and perhaps challenging the views of those who felt patients could tell the difference. This becomes clearer in looking at the main means used by Trusts to identify HCAs and other staff groups.

Uniforms

Most obviously, variously coloured uniforms were used to differentiate occupational groups, and sometimes grades within these groups. However, as a device for identifying HCAs and other staff members, uniforms were problematic. Trusts used variously coloured staff uniforms for different purposes, not only to help patients distinguish between staff groups, but as an internal signalling device and means of fostering Trust values and attitudes. This was illustrated in London, where in justifying the recent introduction of HCA uniforms very similar in colour to those of nurses, the manager showed a greater interest in creating a sense of inclusiveness amongst HCAs than in helping patients tell the differences between nurses and HCAs:

> Manager_London: I would want to make efforts to pull the healthcare assistant body closer to registered nurses. For example, we've recently changed our uniforms and we've taken them out of purple and put them in to blue, which was traditionally a nursing uniform colour, because we felt it would send an important message to healthcare assistants about how integral to the nursing remit they were.

Uniforms were sometimes unevenly taken up across the Trust and wards, in a manner likely to create patient confusion and uncertainty. For example, in London Trust, which, as noted, had recently changed the colour of the HCA uniforms, some continued to wear the old uniform, because it was 'cooler in summer', while a third group wore scrubs because they simply looked 'cool':

> Matron_London: The new uniform, and that's I think a bit of confusion at the moment because some still have the old uniform which used to be like a very light lilac type of colour, but now they're in a light blue, light blue trousers and top.

Confusion in a number of Trusts was likely wrought by the sheer diversity of coloured uniforms on display at any one time in any given ward. Research observation revealed the following uniforms on display during just one ward shift and this does not include a number of roles who wear 'civvies' such as doctors and social workers:

- Ward manager (dark blue top with white piping);
- Band 6 nurse (dark blue top with dark blue lapels);
- Band 5 nurse (dark blue top with pale blue lapels);
- Band 5 newly qualified nurse (first six months: white lapel);
- Matron (maroon top);
- HCA (chocolate/coffee top);
- Bank HCA (all white top);
- Student nurse (white top with thin gold and blue stripes on the collar and arms);
- Phlebotomist (white top with maroon piping);
- Pharmacist (white top with grey piping);
- Occupational therapist (white top with green piping);
- Physiotherapist (white t-shirt);

- Physiotherapist assistant (green t-shirt);
- Domestic (white top with thin vertical blue stripes);
- Ward assistant (pale blue top with white piping);
- Ward clerk (dark blue shirt with a 'spots in squares' pattern);
- Porter (pale blue short sleeved shirt);
- Cardiographer (pale blue top with dark lilac piping).

A similarly long list could have been compiled from any of the observation wards across each of the hospitals. However, it is interesting to point out that on this ward, although the HCA wore a distinctive coloured top (colour now changed), the bank HCA on the shift performing identical tasks wore a white top—the same colour as a student nurse.

There was little hope that patients might make sense of this array of uniforms:

> Ward manager_London: Unless a patient asks about uniforms, we wouldn't mention it.

Badges

Name badges were another means of identification used by Trusts to pursue various ends. They were often designed with certain internal security concerns in mind, limited consideration being given to how easy they were for patients to read:

> Patient_London: They do wear little things but you can't read them … and it's very embarrassing staring at ladies' chests.

There had been some moves away from the use of name badges as a way of reducing infections to the use of free hanging tags, but these appeared no easier for patients to read:

> Matron_London: Unfortunately they [nursing staff] don't have badges anymore, and that's one thing that I can see the infection control side of the things and the health and safety side of things when you're dealing with a patient, that the badges were quite good because people look to see your name and underneath it would say HCA or staff nurse or something … But people have badges to hang round your neck, if someone grabs at it it's a bit, you know, for your own safety really. But I can't read it if I'm, you know, people who can't see very well, if they try and see who this person is but you can't read it from a distance.

Notwithstanding this conflation of purpose in the use of badges, they could have value:

> HCA_South: I always wear my badge, they can tell the difference or you introduce yourself when you go to them, I'm a healthcare assistant, I will be looking after you, I will give you a wash and that. We tell them who we are. I think some knows the different nurses and healthcare assistants.

But again the use of badges could be uneven between HCAs in the same Trust:

> HCA_North: It doesn't help that I've not got a name badge, not my doing again, it were ordered, I were forgotten.

Personal introduction

In some Trusts HCAs were required to formally introduce themselves to new patients. In London, for example, HCAs were routinely expected to make such introductions:

> Ward manager_London: Hopefully they're introducing themselves, that's the main thing ... So when they come in patients are admitted, so they come to the ward and the person who sits to do the admission process, hopefully people are introducing themselves and saying, 'Hello, my name is Sue', or whatever, 'and I'm one of the HCAs on the ward'.

There were many instances where such an introductory routine was followed:

> HCA_London: We always introduce ourselves, like if we had a new patient I would introduce myself, 'I'm a healthcare assistant, my name's [name]','Nice to meet you', that sort of thing. I know for a fact that our relatives are aware of who's trained staff, you know, qualified, if you like, and who's not trained, who's qualified and who isn't.

However, there were few signs that this procedure was seriously enforced, the result being extremely uneven practice:

> HCA_London: Well we don't really introduce ourselves, which you are supposed to do, say, 'Hello, I'm ..., I'm a healthcare assistant, I will look after you.' No, we don't do this, sorry.

In other Trusts, HCAs introductions reflected personal style rather than a Trust protocol. In South an HCA noted:

> HCA_South: I always make it very clear that if I do take a team I actually introduce myself to the patients, they know me anyway, and I explain that I'm not a nurse, I am an HCA. But, you know, if you've got any problems which I can't help you with then I will go and get the nurse.

However, in these cases introduction could sometimes be incomplete. It was common to hear examples of HCAs giving their name but not their position:

> HCA_London: I don't think I do introduce myself as a healthcare assistant, I just think I say I'm [Name].

Indeed, some HCAs knowingly contributed to the confusion, welcoming the patients' misattribution:

> HCA_North: I know I've got a name badge but it's in my pocket at the minute because it fell off ... I think that's quite nice and it's nice of them shouting 'nurse'.

Others would introduce themselves in a reactive rather than a proactive manner: patients would be corrected when they approached an HCA in error, or told about ward roles on request:

> HCA_Midlands: Some of the patients get confused and they'll ask me for some drugs or something, you know, what they needed, tablets, and then I have to explain to them that I'm not a staff nurse. And they'll say 'will you wash me today?' I'll say 'yes, because I'm an auxiliary nurse, not a staff, not a trained, a trained nurse'.

Picture board

A more novel device was the use of a picture board at the entrance to each ward which listed the name and position of staff alongside their photographs. This approach did have some use for patients:

> Patient_North: I mean they had a little plaque up which I found very useful with pictures on at the reception.

However, for less mobile patients, there were clearly limits to its value. Indeed for many patients, particularly those on surgical wards, the first time they would see the photo board would be as they were leaving the ward itself.

The difficulties faced in designing and implementing devices to identify HCAs and other staff members emerged in evidence to suggest that patients often found it difficult to distinguish HCAs. Patients were quite often observed using the generic term 'nurse' to call to any member of the ward team, a point confirmed in interview with many of the nurses and HCAs:

> HCA_Midlands: A lot of the patients, they're not really sure what we are; because only this morning actually a patient thought I was a student nurse. Most of the patients think that you're the tea lady.
> HCA_Midlands: One woman on the ward the other day called the nurse a pharmacist because … honestly, she said, 'Oh there she is, the pharmacist, the one who does the drugs'. And it's like, 'No, that's your staff nurse, that's not your pharmacist'. 'Oh she gives out the drugs', I went, 'Yes, I know, but that's your staff nurse'.

Most tellingly, these difficulties were further reflected in a number of patient focus group comments:

> Patient_North: Care assistants, they are trained to a different level in different things but there's no way of distinguishing it.
> Patient_North: It's extremely difficult because whereas there used to be, you know, different uniforms, they seem to be much more blurred now … and trying to read identification tags is impossible.

In the context of these findings, it is somewhat surprising that in all Trusts the surveys revealed the majority of patients were able to identify the HCA (see Table 9.1). Indeed given the material presented earlier, it is not unreasonable to suggest that these data represent an overstatement of the patients' ability to

Table 9.1 Identifying HCAs (%)

	South	Midlands	North	London	p-value
Able to tell the difference between a nurse and a HCA	66	72	69	58	$\chi^2 = 18.11$, $p < 0.001$
Of those that could tell the difference, how…?[a]					
Told by a HCA	16	11	17	20	
Told by a nurse	19	23	18	21	
Told by other staff	2	6	4	4	
Told by a patient	2	1	3	1	
Told by relative/friend	3	4	3	5	
By the uniform/name badge	70	76	73	67	
Read info. in the hospital	7	6	5	5	
Pictures on notice board	12	11	18	12	
Already knew	20	20	20	12	
Don't know/can't remember	1	2	1	5	
Other	4	2	1	1	

[a]This question is a multi-response format, percentages can exceed 100%

distinguish the HCA. At the same time, the surveys revealed significant differences between the Trusts in this respect: for example, in London, barely half of the surveyed patients could distinguish HCAs, while in Midlands this proportion rose to over three-quarters.

While these survey data suggest that Trusts were more or less successful in impressing staff differences on patients, the effective means of distinguishing HCAs remained fairly standard. Despite concerns raised about uniforms as a way of distinguishing staff roles and grades, they were clearly and by a long way the most common means of identification: around three-quarters of patients who could distinguish did so in this way. There is stronger confirmation of the unevenness of direct communication as a means of conveying staff roles to patients: only around a fifth of patients indicated being directly told about differences by a nurse or HCA. Indeed, in all Trusts, patients are slightly more likely to be told who HCA are, by the nurse rather than the HCA, a finding likely to be explained by nurse control over the admissions process. Moreover, picture or notice boards are confirmed as being of very little value in this respect.

A distinctive relationship

Notwithstanding concerns raised about the ability of patients to distinguish HCAs, it still remains pertinent to ask whether patients developed a distinctive relationship with them. Such a relationship might well develop without patients appreciating the difference between roles given the particular tasks performed by HCAs, their specific demeanour, and orientation towards the patients. The picture to emerge was nuanced, with two patterns, in the main associated with different data sources, emerging: in the first the patient–HCA relationship was distinctive and positive; the second cast greater doubt on the quality of this connection, and implied some patient caution about the role of the HCA. This section describes and then seeks to explain, in turn, these different patterns.

Distinctive and positive

The HCA and nurse interview data revealed a strong and consistent pattern, suggesting that patients did indeed have a very particular relationship with HCAs. In general, HCAs were seen as being closer to patients than nurses. This closeness was presented in various ways: patients were more likely to view the HCAs as a 'friend' or confidant; they had a better rapport with HCAs; and they found it easier to confide in them. Such features of the patient–HCA relationship were consistently mentioned across all Trusts:

> Matron_Midlands: The patients see them [HCAs] as the main people that they see. It's not very often you'd hear a complaint that's about the healthcare assistants.
> Ward manager_London: [HCAs] probably develop a more substantial relationship with the patients compared to the staff nurse who I think is quite busy doing lots of different things. I just think because people are giving direct care nursing assistant-wise that the relationships might be a bit sort of more developed.
> Matron_North: [Patients] pick up they're different. And sometimes a patient will wait until they see an HCA to ask them something rather than bother a qualified nurse.
> Sister_South: Support workers have a more open, friendly sort of, like a friend's rapport. I'm generalising here, there are always exceptions, and I'm not saying that doesn't happen with trained staff but because trained staff perhaps don't always have quite such a long hands-on involvement, because of doing medicines and doing other things, they probably see the healthcare assistants more and so the relationship does develop differently. And I think sometimes the patients can see the support workers as actually doing more for them than the trained staff.

The closeness of the patient–HCA relationship was confirmed by some of the observational material. If the patient was seeking a 'friend', this was seen almost invariably to be the HCA:

> Field note_North (Medical): There is one instance where a patient spends a long time explaining her worries and fears in the observee's [HCA] presence. Observee comes across as a good listener.
> Field note_London (Surgical): The observee [an HCA] appeared to be the ward mascot – many patients even those not in his bay knew his name and called his name as he passed by. He was very chatty and did seem to have time to sit and chat, listen with patients. During a long wash a patient was telling him in some detail about her recent

bowel movements. He spent time comforting a particularly dependent patient and helping her feed. The observee was valued by patients as a consequence of his happy demeanour, accessibility and willingness to help. So, early in the shift he sorted out the battery of a patient's hearing aid to which she replied 'my hero', and various other comments from patients suggested the observee's value. 'He's a very happy lad to have around and he's very competent, nothing is too much trouble for him.'

Most striking was the support for a distinctive and positive patient–HCA relationship provided by the survey data on what we labelled 'caring behaviours'. Asked whether they find it difficult or easy to deal with various sort of patients, HCAs in all four Trusts found it easier to enact caring behaviours than nurses (see Table 9.2). The difference was particularly striking in Midlands, where the mean score for HCA and nurses were respectively 3.50 and 3.26. But in general HCAs found it easier than nurses to deal with patients who were:

- deeply upset;
- verbally abusive; and
- confused.

These data need to be treated with some caution. As self-report questions, HCAs and nurses were approaching them from very different perspectives. Most obviously nurses with their formal medical and clinical training might arguably be more sensitive to the complexity of dealing with difficult situations and patients than the HCA. However, these survey data on caring behaviours did find some support from our observations, highlighting instances where the HCA appeared to be particularly effective in dealing with such matters:

> Field note_North (Medical): A patient came onto the ward during the night and [during observation] had three major episodes of bewilderment, anxiety and raw emotion. Both of the latter times saw the observee [HCA] crouch down on her knees to maintain eye level whilst holding his hands as she listened and tried to centre the patient. The second time took six minutes, which was a considerable period of time given the speed of ward life. The latter episode was also noteworthy as the observee joined a Band 5 after she had been largely ineffective in her attempt and stayed sitting down during this period almost entirely redundant as the observee took over.

This greater HCA sensitivity to difficult situations was also reflected in some of the patients' comments:

> Patient_South: There were two girls [HCAs], three girls actually at [Hospital] who were absolutely excellent. They were fantastic and you felt, I mean one took me for a shower after my operation, a couple days after my operation, and I just felt she'd got all the time in the world for me and it was, that does make a difference when you, because you've got so many worries at that point.

In seeking to explain this distinctive and positive relationship between patients and HCAs, a relationship which suggests that HCAs were not only

Table 9.2 Caring behaviours (mean score)

How difficult or easy do you find it to:	South		Midlands		North		London		p-value	
	HCAs	Nurses	HCAs	Nurses	HCAs	Nurses	HCAs	Nurses	HCAs	Nurses
... develop a close relationship with a verbally abusive patient	2.72	2.32	2.84	2.52	2.73	2.46	2.76	2.49	$F = 0.516$, $p = 0.671$	$F = 1.76$, $p = 0.153$
... calm a patient who is very stressed about their medical condition	3.36	3.37	3.45	3.41	3.47	3.58	3.29	3.40	$F = 1.30$, $p = 0.274$	$F = 2.08$, $p = 0.101$
... develop a close relationship with a patient whose background is different from your own	3.72	3.67	3.80	3.68	3.93	3.78	3.83	3.80	$F = 2.22$, $p = 0.085$	$F = 1.33$, $p = 0.264$
... cheer up a patient who is deeply upset about an aspect of their stay	3.78	3.54	3.93	3.68	3.94	3.73	3.99	3.71	$F = 2.06$, $p = 0.105$	$F = 2.21$, $p = 0.086$
... develop a close relationship with a confused patient	3.32	2.92	3.46	3.04	3.50	3.21	3.22	3.02	$F = 2.73$, $p = 0.043$	$F = 2.48$, $p = 0.060$
SCALE: Caring behaviours[a]	**3.38**	**3.16**	**3.50**	**3.26**	**3.51**	**3.35**	**3.42**	**3.28**	**$F = 1.72$, $p = 0.161$**	**$F = 2.72$, $p = 0.044$**

[a] Two-way ANOVA main effects: Role, $F = 27.49$, $p < 0.001$; Trust, $F = 4.03$, $p = 0.007$

closer to patients but better able to deal with the difficult cases, a number of possible explanatory factors emerged.

Tasks and time

The first related to the tasks performed by HCAs. As Figure 6.1 has highlighted, HCAs do spend a much higher proportion of their shift providing direct and indirect patient care. The provision of such intimate care might afford the HCA more time with the patient allowing a closer relationship to develop. This link between tasks and a distinctive patient–HCA connection was consistently stressed:

> HCA_North: There was one woman and she was really conscious like about getting washed and she said, 'I don't want anyone else to do it but you, you come in in the morning and you help me'. And I was like 'oh I will', and she were like 'I don't want anyone else', things like that. But I think they talk to me more because I'm there more.
>
> Nurse_Midlands: Because they spend more time with them [patients], because most of the time they're probably helping them with the washing while we're like doing our tablets or doing bloods and stuff, they're doing like the little things ... And like they'll [HCAs] come and speak to them [patients] and sit with them and talk to them, and then they'll go over the whole ward.
>
> Nurse_London: Because the HCAs are probably doing sometimes more hands-on nursing than us, they probably are the ones that are going to get to know them, they're the ones that are going to have the little chats with them and, you know, while they're washing them and that sort of thing.
>
> HCA_South: We have a lot more to do with the personal care normally and we've got more time to sort of actually talk to them rather than the nurses usually dash in with medication and dash out again. They say 'oh I'll see you about two o'clock with your next medication' and they, because they've got too much to do, you know, that we can actually, when we finished all the personal care, just sit down and talk to someone, if you're doing twenty minutes [a bed wash].

The other side of this coin sees the nurse as being driven away from the bedside by other tasks and less available to develop a close relationship with patient:

> Nurse_London: I don't think the trained nurses have so much patient contact because they've got the admissions and discharges and all that paperwork side to do then, and then I think there's a lot of other things they have to sort out, the District Nurse things.
>
> HCA_South: We have far more patient contact than staff nurses because we're there, because they take, you know, we do everything for these patients. You know, the staff nurses, if they're on a team they've got fifteen other people who they're busy, you know, coordinating with the doctors what the treatment's going to be or what drugs they're going to have, so they're not always actually with the patient but HCAs are, you see, because we're constantly on the ward doing that, that's what, you know, that's what we do.

Most significantly, patients often saw the HCA as more accessible, more available to talk to and confide in:

Patient_North: I think they (HCAs) were a very important part of the staff, yes ... the nurses can be getting on with more important stuff, can't they?

Patient_North: If you want something doing ask an [HCA], they will do it a lot quicker than the full-time nurses.

Patient_North: They seemed to have a bit more time to chat than the professionals do. Does that make sense? ... and you need that on a ward, you need somebody that's happy to chat, you know ... because then you become a friendly atmosphere ... until somebody starts to chat, you're all isolated.

Patient_North: One [HCA], she was like right chatty, she was nice, you know, she'd come over, she'd say alright, time to get your bed changed and ... whilst she was doing it she would talk, while he sat on the chair she'd, you know, have a little chat with him as well.

Patient_London: The ones in [hospital name], I must admit, would come and talk to you while they were taking your blood pressure or temperature or whatever it may be, at least they would talk to you. The nurses didn't seem to have time to talk to you.

Patient_London: There was just a slight sense they had a little bit more time, they weren't quite so rushed.

Patient_London: I want somebody who ... has got the common sense, unlike some of the nurses, to actually as she's moving away, to draw the ... curtain as she went away ... and I think the healthcare assistant was always that much more focused on the person through no ... deliberate act of their own happened to be in a hospital bed.

Patient_London: They do the extra things, don't they, the little things ... one day my daughter didn't come up, and she [HCA] said, 'Oh, you haven't had your paper ... I'll nip down in my break and get you a paper'. I mean something little like that ... but it meant a lot.

Patient_Midlands: I would agree that the [HCAs] have got more time ... they made you feel more at ease on the ward ... they're one of us.

The nature of the role

It has been suggested that the status of the HCA might also make it easier for the patient to engage with them rather than the nurse or other care professionals. This found some support in the views of nurses and HCAs, who stressed that patients sometimes found it difficult to approach the nurse, viewing the HCA as a less intimidating point of contact:

Ward manager_North: Some patients don't like to bother staff nurses because they think they're busy doing other things and they might be horrified if I'm doing a bed bath. A senior sister doing that, and they're like I can't believe you're doing a bed bath. And there's a culture thing that they just don't expect that rank to be actually hands-on, whereas they would probably expect the healthcare assistant to be doing more, more of that role.

Matron_North: They see the HCAs out in the bays more actually doing things with the patients more than they would see a qualified nurse, so I think that they feel that they're more approachable to ask. For things like a fruit bowl or whatever, you know, they don't want to bother the qualified nurse, they'll ask the healthcare for it.

HCA_London: Sometimes the patients find it a bit difficult to talk to the staff nurses, you know if they use their lingo like 'You've got to have your TTOs'. And then they'll wait for us to come along with our brown uniforms and ask 'What's a TTO?' and we can explain.

Matron_Midlands: If you've not been exposed to healthcare, to actually come in and be a patient is really scary and I think the person that you'll approach will be the [HCA]. They're the person that's around, they certainly haven't got that air of 'oh I don't want to ask the consultant, he might shout at me!' People still think that, and that's why it's a very, very essential role.

Again it is striking that this view of the HCA as more accessible given their status is echoed in patient remarks:

Patient_Midlands: Sometimes you feel as though you can ask an [HCA] if they're passing by or whatever, but a nurse, you're a bit more reserved because you think they've something more important that they should be doing.

The nature of the post holder

A final possible explanation for the closeness of the patient–HCA relationship lies in the background characteristics of the HCA. We have argued that the kinds of people who become HCAs might more readily relate to patients than some nurses, and might bring with them the tacit skills to do so. Attention has already be drawn to the HCA who, given her ethnic background, was able to translate the patient's wishes on behalf of the nurses. More generally, patients remarked on this implied empathy between the HCA and the patient:

Patient_Midlands: You could have a laugh and a joke with those in the brown uniforms [the HCAs], but those in the blue uniforms [nurses] you've got to watch your 'Ps' and 'Qs'.

Patient_Midlands: Auxiliaries, they're one of us. They're just a person like us. They come along and say 'You alright?'… They're one of you and you can talk to them.

Indeed, another example emerged during observation, of the HCAs' ability to draw upon their background to link to the patient:

Field note_Midlands (Medical): This HCA is an example of the bridging link that HCAs have with the community. She found it very easy to talk to patients, find out details about them and to try and make connections with them. One new patient on the ward meeting her for the first time found out that he was born two doors from her husband and was friends with her husband's brother. The entire interaction took less than two minutes but the value to the patient was noticeable, his demeanour changed immediately and each time the HCA was back on the bay he was keen to explore further connections and nostalgia. For elderly and scared patients such connections must make a real qualitative difference to their hospital experience.

More cautious and uncertain

The presentation of the HCA–patient relationship as distinctive and positive, with patients able to develop a closer connection by virtue of the tasks performed by the HCA, the nature of the role, and its post holders, needs to be tempered in some respects. There was evidence to indicate that patients were somewhat more cautious and uncertain in their relationship with HCAs. There were signs to suggest that elements of the less positive scenario held sway, with patient concerns about the implications of the HCA role for the quality of care they received.

This less positive scenario was manifest in a numbers of ways. In part, it was reflected in the very different HCA and nurse perceptions of the distinctive contribution made by the HCA. Our co-production scale, which explicitly sought to evaluate the particular contribution of HCAs, asked both groups whether HCAs were more likely to engage with and notice concerns amongst patients. As Table 9.3 indicates, in all four Trusts, nurses viewed HCAs as less likely to sensitively address patients than themselves; while HCAs in turn felt that it was they rather than the nurses who dealt sensitively with patients. This is further illustrated in Figure 9.1 which notes that while almost three-quarters of HCAs 'agree' or 'strongly agree' that compared to nurses they 'take time to listen to patients when they need to talk', barely a quarter of nurses concurred with this view.

These are findings which overlap somewhat with the discussion in the last chapter, which suggested that nurses were rather more grudging about the contribution made by HCAs in the survey than in interview: it will be recalled that in interview nurses were quite fulsome in their praise for the distinctive HCA contribution to patient care. In the current context, it is a finding which connects to a view found in some of the Trusts that there was nothing intrinsic to the HCA role or its post holders which enabled them to develop a particularly close relationship with patients. Those holding this view were more inclined to stress the tasks performed by HCAs which allowed them to develop such a relationship. If nurses had the same time to undertake direct care, they also would establish such a link with patients:

> Senior nurse_North: [HCAs] generally have most probably a closer relationship because they're more in the bays and more to be seen I think, to be honest. And that's the odd thing, you know, when you strip someone off and they reveal all and the conversation starts flowing, but *I can't actually say if a staff nurse did the same thing, I don't think there's any difference* [emphasis added].
> Ward manager_Midlands: I don't think it's a case that they [HCAs] can offer things that nurses can't, I think they've just got that more time at the bedside than a trained nurse has.

Table 9.3 Co-production value (mean score)

Compared to nurses, HCAs are more likely to:[a]	South		Midlands		North		London		p-value	
	HCAs	Nurses	HCAs	Nurses	HCAs	Nurses	HCAs	Nurses	HCAs	Nurses
… notice when patients are in discomfort	3.54	2.51	3.67	2.62	3.34	2.86	3.93	2.54	$F = 7.20$, $p < 0.001$	$F = 3.45$, $p = 0.016$
… show concern when patients complain	3.63	2.50	3.66	2.57	3.34	2.75	3.97	2.45	$F = 8.22$, $p < 0.001$	$F = 2.22$, $p = 0.085$
… talk to patients in a warm friendly manner	3.81	2.85	3.65	2.87	3.35	3.16	3.91	2.70	$F = 7.90$, $p < 0.001$	$F = 4.27$, $p = 0.005$
… be told by patients about their worries and concerns	3.83	2.71	3.81	2.58	3.64	2.98	4.08	2.54	$F = 4.37$, $p = 0.005$	$F = 5.06$, $p = 0.002$
… explain what they are doing when working with patients	3.67	2.49	3.67	2.45	3.45	2.64	3.80	2.34	$F = 2.74$, $p = 0.043$	$F = 1.89$, $p = 0.130$
… take time to listen to patients when they need to talk	4.02	2.78	3.94	2.74	3.69	3.01	3.95	2.61	$F = 3.34$, $p = 0.019$	$F = 3.00$, $p = 0.030$
SCALE: Co-production value[b]	**3.75**	**2.64**	**3.73**	**2.64**	**3.47**	**2.90**	**3.94**	**2.53**	**$F = 7.18$, $p < 0.001$**	**$F = 4.20$, $p = 0.006$**

[a] For nurses the original wording and scoring have been reversed so that all results are from the point of view of HCAs to ease interpretation of the data

[b] Two-way ANOVA main effects: Role, $F = 428.28$, $p < 0.001$; Trust, $F = 0.18$, $p = 0.911$

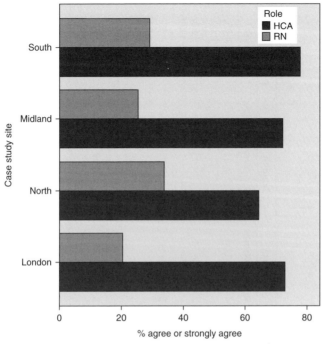

Figure 9.1 HCAs are more likely to listen to patients[a] by role (%)[b]. ([a] For nurses the original wording and scoring have been reversed to aid interpretation.[b] % is those who agreed or strongly agreed with the statement.)

Equally, if not more noteworthy, the patient survey findings also encouraged a more qualified view of the HCA–patient relationship than apparent from the patient focus groups. Table 9.4 indicates that patients rated the care received both from HCAs and nurses extremely highly; however, across all Trusts the mean scores are significantly higher for nurses than HCAs. Looking at the specific items on this scale, it is particularly apparent that when it came to answering questions about care and when seeking someone to confide in, the nurse scores were significantly higher than for HCAs. While, as noted, these findings are slightly at odds with the main tenor of the qualitative analysis, they nonetheless throw up some patient and relative concerns about the HCA role. This is sometimes apparent in the disrespect shown to HCAs:

> Nurse_Midlands: If it's gone like visiting time, if a nurse can say it's end of visiting, then the patient families will get up and go, but if it's an [HCA] that say it it's 'who does she think she's talking to', you know, that kind of thing.
> HCA_London: Sometimes I feel that as HCAs we're belittled, we're treated like second class citizens. Which again hasn't happened between staff, but I definitely feel that through kind of sometimes some patients' interactions with us or the sort of patients'

Table 9.4 Difference between care given by HCAs versus nurses (mean score)

Statements: a	South		Midlands		North		London		p-value	
	HCAs	Nurses	HCAs	Nurses	HCAs	Nurses	HCAs	Nurses	HCAs	Nurses
[...] were willing to listen to what I had to say	4.01	4.21	4.11	4.33	4.03	4.04	3.99	4.01	$F = 0.55$, $p = 0.651$	$F = 4.85$, $p = 0.002$
When [...] answered questions about my care I was able to understand them	3.91	4.21	4.01	4.21	3.91	4.11	3.96	4.13	$F = 0.56$, $p = 0.644$	$F = 0.86$, $p = 0.460$
I was able to confide in [...]	3.62	3.93	3.90	4.19	3.61	3.99	3.61	3.92	$F = 3.21$, $p = 0.023$	$F = 3.12$, $p = 0.025$
I was treated with respect and dignity by [...]	4.24	4.28	4.36	4.43	4.21	4.23	4.14	4.18	$F = 2.72$, $p = 0.044$	$F = 2.51$, $p = 0.058$
SCALE: Patient reported care[b]	**3.96**	**4.15**	**4.11**	**4.30**	**3.96**	**4.09**	**3.95**	**4.09**	**$F = 2.00$, $p = 0.113$**	**$F = 2.93$, $p = 0.033$**

[a] [...] are used to indicate where the term 'Healthcare assistants' or 'Nurses' was used in the statement. Patient respondents who had previously stated that they could tell the difference between HCAs and nurses rated each statement for both staff groups

[b] Repeated measures ANOVA: $F = 37.77$, $p < 0.001$

views of us as HCAs. But I do feel like that, we're treated as a second class citizen in the role that we do.

Indeed, this disrespect assumes an even stronger form when patients are unwilling to engage with HCAs:

HCA_Midlands: I've got some people that like they don't even want to talk to you because you're not really, you're only an auxiliary sort of thing. And, but some of them will, they'll think well, you know, I might sort of ask you a few questions, do you think you could help me with this and, so it depends on the person really.

In a more benign form, it was suggested that some patients just felt more assured by talking to a nurse rather than an HCA:

Senior nurse_South: If somebody's not feeling very well and I think they're a bit more reassured by the darker uniform.
Sister_South: If the patient thinks they're not a trained nurse they'll say oh you're, you know, someone will say 'well you're not a trained nurse, I don't want you' … I've noticed that sometimes in the past where, you know, you're not trained, I don't want you doing that or something, you know, that might happen on the flipside.

This finds some confirmation in the views of patients, who were more inclined to approach the nurse rather than the HCA when they had more technical, clinical questions to ask:

Patient_Midlands: I mean if I had any big questions to ask, it was always the nurses. But I did find the [HCAs] were nice and friendly and if you'd had a long night with no sleep … they was the first face you saw and they sort of put your mind at rest really.
Patient_London: If I did have any questions of a … medical nature, I would generally want to put them to the sister … I would have been more or less happy with a nurse … but I wouldn't have been happy putting those questions to a healthcare assistant.

The identification of two patterns of patient–HCA relations—one assuming a distinctive and positive form and the other a more uncertain and cautious one—represents something of a conundrum. Certainly it encourages a search for reasons as to why these patterns might coexist, with a number of possible explanations worth exploring.

Methodology

The different patterns might be related to the research methods used. In the main, the distinctive and positive pattern of patient–HCA relations emerged from the interview, focus group, and observational data, while the more uncertain and cautious one was found in the survey material. The former techniques, all involving the presence of a researcher, might encourage a 'softer' portrayal of patient–HCA relations than the former self administered techniques. Some care is needed, however, in proposing such an explanation: there was not a straightforward or hard and fast correlation between research method and pattern of patient–HCA relations. Our survey data on caring behaviours pointed to a distinctive and positive relationship between patients and HCAs, while there was considerable interview and focus group material to support a more cautious and uncertain relationship.

Complementarity

Reliance on a methodological rationale for a disconnect in findings is significantly weakened if a plausible story can be presented to explain the coexistence of the two patterns. Thus, it might be argued that these patterns are complementary rather than in tension with another. The findings lend plausibility to a narrative which suggests that when it comes to routine and ongoing direct care, patients do form a distinctive and positive relationship with HCAs, but when it comes to more technical, clinical issues they are more inclined to approach and seek a relationship with the registered nurse.

Contradictions

Another, equally plausible, story suggests that patients might well hold contradictory views of HCA at the same time. This is different to the previous story, in that it does not claim the two patterns are necessarily compatible. Given the incomplete knowledge held by the patient about the HCA role, it is conceivable that views oscillate in non-rational ways, or sit uneasily alongside one another, with the patient unable to form a clear and a decisive view of the HCA.

Selectivity

The most ambitious explanation for the coexistence of the two patterns lies in the possibility that patients draw selectively on their memories of engagement with HCAs. More specifically, our findings suggest that patient contact with ward staff, and particularly HCAs, took various forms. This contact could be brief and fleeting. Indeed despite the impressions of our stakeholders that HCAs spent considerable time with patients, particularly in the provision of direct patient care, our observation data suggest that in practice this contact was very short. Figure 9.2, based upon these observational data, reveals the average time spent by an HCA in undertaking a direct task was barely more than five minutes. Certainly this was slightly longer than the time taken by a nurse on such tasks, but only by a minute or so.

In addition to this fleeting contact, there were more sporadic instances of sustained and intense HCA contact with patients. These instances were again mainly picked up in observation. Some attention has already been given to

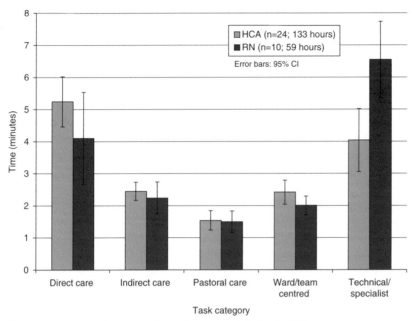

Figure 9.2 Average time per task—HCAs versus RNs (early shift).

these episodes, but it is worth quoting another at length to highlight the impact such contact with HCA might have upon the patient:

> Field note_Midlands (Medical): The patient was in his 50s, 24 stone and almost seven foot tall and had developed a spinal abscess that burst and left him partially paralysed during a previous stay in hospital. He had returned to the ward with exceptionally bad leg ulcers and renal failure. Nurses were heard to complain that the patient had kept up to four staff busy for over five hours during the previous day's late shift and at one point been verbally abusive such that an adjoining bed had to be cleared. After lunch the HCA was between tasks and took the opportunity to approach this patient. The HCA made an introduction, sat down and then said very little, letting the patient slowly engage and talk. The patient began to open up and talk about his life before the paralysis. He went on to reveal that aside from his medical condition he was very upset about his hiccups that were uncomfortable, had been going on for six weeks and which the patient believed made him sound like he had a speech impediment. The patient described how this was the first time he'd talked about his hiccups since being admitted to the ward. The patient thanked the HCA, and shortly after ventured out of the bay on his wheelchair for the first time since being admitted and calmly discussed his situation at the nurses' station. The HCA later returned to help the patient onto a commode: the patient remarked 'I'm glad to have met you today'. Towards the end of the shift two senior nurses were overheard discussing how the patient had changed for the better.

This is an example which not only provides some further support for the important role played by the HCA in dealing with difficult situations and patients, but in the context of the current discussion, highlights instances of deep and affecting patient engagement with the HCA. It is suggested that such engagement, when set aside the more fleeting routine contact with patients, helps account for the contrasting views held by these patients about the HCA: the typically brief contact is being drawn upon by patients in their somewhat cautious views of HCAs, while the isolated instances of more sustained and affecting contact are relied on by patients in assessing the HCAs' contribution as distinctive and positive.

Does it matter?

In assessing 'bottom line' outcomes, the study sought to explore the link between the patients' ability to identify HCAs and the quality of their care experience. It has been noted that views amongst stakeholders varied as to whether patients could distinguish the HCA, and in this section we consider whether this matters anyway.

The value of patients being able to distinguish HCAs from other members of the ward team is partly contingent. Patients are sometime too ill to care greatly about any distinction between staff members, and as implied earlier, not concerned as long as care is 'adequate'. There were, in addition, some who felt that it was not even desirable for patients to distinguish: patients should be comfortable in approaching any member of the nursing team in a seamless way:

> Ward manager_North: I want to know that [patients] can speak to anyone and the confidence that the patient has to be able to speak to somebody who's qualified and somebody who's not qualified in the same way, rather than going 'well I can't speak to her because she doesn't know anything about it and she's not qualified', and it stigmatises somebody who's not qualified to somebody who is, to be fair.

At the same time, our qualitative data suggested the plausibility of an association between the ability to distinguish the HCA and the quality of the patient experience. General uncertainty about what is happening to a patient is likely to contribute to a feeling of confusion and disorientation, while more tangibly, given some ongoing demarcations on who does what on the ward, knowing precisely who to approach with certain questions and requests is likely to have a profound impact on physical and mental well-being. The importance of being able to identify the right member of staff was reflected in a number of patient comments:

> Patient_London: I was in a lot of pain and I would often ask for pain relief and it would be a HCA and she, 'You'll have to wait a minute because I have to go and ask

sister … and get it signed off' … And I didn't feel frustrated, I felt frustrated with the system.

Patient_South: Part of my [hospital] experience and the bad part of the experience I had now I can see because I was asking the wrong questions to the wrong people, because I didn't understand the difference. So I was probably asking a healthcare assistant something that he or she wasn't qualified really to deal with, and done their best to accommodate me but didn't deliver my expectation and made me more frustrated. So I think this comes around that the communication of really understanding who's doing what roles and where their roles stop in terms of qualification and the next role starts, because that awareness I think helps the patient as much as it does help the system.

Indeed this inability to distinguish could have knock-on effects: the frustration and sometimes anger of the patient being conveyed to the HCA:

HCA_London: Sometimes it can be difficult because sometimes the patient can be very horrible to you. Sometimes they would see you and they rung the bell and you goes to them and you say, 'What can I do for you now, Mrs So-and-so?' And she said, 'Oh I'm in so much pain and I would like some pain, strong pain tablet.' And then you says to them, 'OK, I'll get the nurse to give it to you, because I can't give it to you'. And then you go and you tell it to the nurse, maybe the nurse is caught up into something, maybe the other nurse is on her break, maybe the one nurse is at Theatre or something, but you know you tell it to one. So he says, 'OK, as soon as I'm finished I'll go and give it'. And then that patient would see you passing again and they ring the bell, and you go back to them and they says to you, 'Oh I told you I just wanted a tablet, medication, and you walking around, I'm having so much pain, you know', and then they started to talk. And those are the patients who, you know, write about us.

The patient survey findings strongly endorse the relationship between HCA identification and care quality. As Table 9.5 indicates, across each Trust the result is the same: patients who can tell the difference between HCAs and nurses report a significantly more positive hospital experience. Even when controlling for the impact of other survey variables that may impact on the relationship—patient age, gender, ethnicity, length of stay, frequency of visits, or number of wards stayed on—there remains an additional positive and significant relationship between patients' knowledge about staff role differences

Table 9.5 Overall rating of care by knowledge of staff role differences (mean score)

	South	Midlands	North	London	p-value
Patient could tell the difference between HCAs and nurses:					
Yes	3.83	4.03	3.60	3.71	$F = 52.20$, $p < 0.001$
No	3.59	3.50	3.15	3.35	

and their reported assessment of care (Change in $R^2 = 0.04$, change in $F = 59.88$, $p < 0.001$).

The message is clear: while Trusts are at best only moderately successful in helping patients distinguish between HCAs and nurses, there are benefits to be had from making sure that patients are not left to deduce differences by uniforms alone, but are actively informed by the staff themselves and/or through other means.

Summary

The consequence of the HCA role for the patient was one of the key issues for our research: how patients view and engage with HCAs is clearly central to the patient experience, and, as a result, to the concerns of policymakers and practitioners at national and Trust level. It was suggested that these consequences might assume different forms: a positive scenario where patients were able to draw upon the HCA as a less intimidating and more accessible form of care; a negative scenario where the low status and unregulated nature of the role might generate care quality concerns amongst patients; or a complementary, perhaps contradictory, combination of these negative and positive scenarios.

In exploring these outcomes, the study drew upon an unusually rich database: the views of HCAs, nurses, and, most importantly, patients were available through interviews, surveys, and focus groups, underpinned by extensive observation of HCA—and nurse—patient contact. The picture to emerge was a complex and nuanced one, with a disconnect between the data and the views of different stakeholders. It was a picture perhaps closest to the third option: the positive and negative scenarios sitting uneasily alongside one another.

The patient–HCA relationship was addressed by considering three questions: whether patients could distinguish HCAs from other members of the nursing team; whether HCAs had a distinctive relationship with patients; and whether distinguishing the HCA mattered from a patient perspective. Distinguishing HCAs from other members of the ward team, particularly nurses, was difficult for patients. A significant minority of surveyed patients indicated they could not identify HCAs and given the problems highlighted with Trust attempts to communicate staff differences—uniforms, picture boards, introductions, badges—this was likely to be an underestimate. This patient difficulty in spotting the HCA mattered. We found strong evidence that those patients able to correctly distinguish had a better care experience, a plausible relationship given the likely patient frustration in seeking care from inappropriate staff members.

The bulk of the chapter concentrated on the nature of the patient–HCA relationship. The findings suggested the coexistence of a distinctive and positive set of relations with more cautious and uncertain ones. The former pattern was founded on the added value brought by the HCA role to the patient experience: what has been referred to throughout this book as the role's co-production function. The HCA was viewed as being closer to the patient than other members of the ward team, establishing the HCA as a unique source of patient comfort, 'friendship', and close care. Such a contribution found its most potent support in survey data suggesting that the HCA found it easier than the nurse to deal with difficult patients and situations, a finding supported by a number of observed incidents. This pattern was variously linked to the tasks performed by the HCAs—the more direct care tasks undertaken by HCAs providing a more sustained and intimate contact with patients—and to features of the role and its post holders, which provided patients with a more accessible source of care.

The more cautious and uncertain patient response to HCAs was somewhat at odds with this distinctive and positive pattern. It was partly reflected in competing HCA and registered nurse views as to which group most sensitively engaged with patients, but more significantly in survey results indicating that patients often preferred to deal with nurses than HCAs.

The chapter explored the reasons why such contrasting patterns might coexist. The respective patterns were supported by different sorts of data, the positive pattern had a slightly stronger basis in the qualitative material, and the more cautious pattern in the quantitative data, prompting consideration of whether different methods encouraged 'softer' or 'harder' views on the patient–HCA relationship. There were, however, a number of plausible narratives which might account for these coexisting patterns. One suggested that they might well be complementary, patients preferring to deal with different members of the ward team depending on the issue at stake. Another was founded on the view that patients might draw selectively on their different experiences of HCAs, the more cautious pattern being linked to the routine fleeting contact with HCAs, the positive pattern associated with sporadic instances of more intense and affecting engagement with HCAs.

Issues for reflection

The findings in this part of the report suggest the need for Trusts to consider the following in respect to consequences for patients:

- Ensuring that patients can distinguish between HCAs and other members of the ward team: in particular explaining to patients the contribution made by different ward roles, so allowing them to know who to approach for what.

- Acknowledging and leveraging the distinctive relationship HCAs are able to develop with patients: this includes HCAs finding it easier to deal with certain difficult types of patient than nurses; being able to get closer to patients; and patients finding it easier to relate to HCAs.
- The ongoing preference of patients to deal with nurses rather than HCAs on some issues.

Chapter 10

Summary and conclusions

For good or ill, the healthcare assistant's time has now come. A long-standing feature of the nursing workforce, it has been thrust centre stage by a combination of recent developments. The HCA is, however, nervously positioned in the spotlight, as policymakers and practitioners at national, regional, and Trust levels remain uncertain about the role they should play. As 'casting directors' these policymakers and practitioners have been torn between, on the one hand, using the HCA as a flexible, relatively low-cost resource, increasingly important in times of financial constraint, and on the other, advancing a quality and safety agenda which questions, perhaps baulks, at the use of the HCA in these ways. It is a dilemma enacted in the full glare of debate about the regulation of the HCA role. As the professional nursing establishment lines up behind calls for tighter regulation, bolstered by an ever increasing number of high-profile cases of healthcare failure, linked with varying degrees of explicitness to concerns about skill mix, governments have prevaricated, and only slowly moved towards a regulatory response.

These debates about the place, role, and regulation of the HCA have been played out on an extremely patchy and fragile evidence base. Policymakers and practitioner engagement with the role has been founded upon a very limited appreciation of those who undertake the role, the form taken by the role, and how the role impacts on key stakeholders. The primary purpose of this book was to address these issues, and in so doing help ensure that policymaking and practice as it relates to the HCA are more informed and considered.

A healthcare assistant role working alongside, often in support of the registered nurse was presented as a common feature of healthcare workforces in developed and less developed countries. It was a role, however, which assumed different forms, a testament to the choices available to national policymakers, but also an indication of how deeply embedded the role might be in the broader political economy of the country's healthcare system. In Britain, developments over the last 20 years or so had not only propelled the HCA role to the main support for the registered nurse, but opened up a much more extended space for its performance. Traditionally performing in an auxiliary capacity away from the bedside, the HCA had increasingly taken on activities which overlapped with those of the registered nurse.

Against this backdrop, policymakers and practitioners in Britain have drawn upon the HCA role to pursue various objectives. It was seen as a role which could act as a relief—removing routine tasks from nurses; as a substitute—replacing the registered nurse in the provision of some core nursing tasks; as an apprentice—providing a future supply of assistant practitioners (APs) and nurses; and as a co-producer—enhancing care quality by bringing distinctive capabilities to bear on the care process.

These public policy goals were, however, based on a number of heroic assumptions about: the strategic orientation of Trusts on workforce issues; the background of those taking up the HCA role; the shape and structure of the HCA post; and to its consequences for the post holders themselves, the nurses they worked with, and the patients they cared for. The research literature on the HCA had provided important insights into many of these issues: on the personal characteristics of HCAs; on the malleability of the role; on its degraded character; and on the ambiguity of nurses towards it. Nonetheless, this literature was presented as diffuse in its focus, under-theorized and methodologically uneven.

The research presented in this book sought to address four questions which derived from policymaker and practitioner assumptions about the potential use of the HCA role: Are HCAs considered by Trusts as a strategic resource? Who are HCAs? What do they do? How does the role impact on post holders, nurses, and patients?

Our analysis was based on a framework which suggested that the answers to these questions might well be influenced by a range of contingent factors. These contingent influences, which shaped our research approach, included:

- Local labour markets as well as Trust policy and practice, encouraging the selection of four case study Trusts drawn from different regions of the country (following a wider range of regional Trust interviews);

- Clinical division, with consideration being given to the role in general medical and general surgical wards within each Trust;

- Individual agency, with a concomitant attempt to examine the relationship between HCA backgrounds, action, and the shape as well as the consequences of the role;

- Data source, with qualitative and quantitative research methods being adopted in the form of interviews, observation, focus groups, and surveys; and

- Stakeholder perspectives, with material collected from HCAs, nurses, and patients.

This final chapter is divided into three parts: the first summarizes the findings as they relate to the four core questions; the second returns to the policy goals and assumptions, assessing the evidence base for them; and the third looks to future developments both in terms of the HCA role and further research related to it.

Broadly, the findings presented suggest the standardizing influence of the NHS on the HCA role: important similarities can be found across the four Trusts in who fills the role, its shape, and consequences. However, against this backdrop, contingent influences were found to produce variation along these dimensions. Clinical division emerges as an influence on some aspect of the HCA role, but more important were difference between Trusts. These Trust differences suggested the effect of local labour markets as well as of corporate policies and practices on the role. The scope for individual agency in shaping the role within the context of these structural constraints remained muted, but still present, with personal background linked to some job crafting. Different data sources often aligned with one another, confirming the validity of findings, yet there were disconnects, for example, between the quantitative and qualitative data on how nurses and patients viewed the HCA. Moreover, a shared view on aspects of the HCA role could not detract from differences of opinion on others, for example, differences of view between HCAs and nurses on who performs certain care tasks. Such differences suggest some contradictions and ambiguities in the nature and consequences of the HCA role, with the need for some care in how the role is used and viewed by policymakers and practitioners at different levels within secondary healthcare.

An overview of findings

Strategic orientations

While Trust executive directors and senior managers routinely expressed the organizational value of the HCA, there was little to suggest a strong strategic orientation to the role in terms of a planned and considered approach linking its use to the pursuit of corporate objectives. This is not to detract from standard statements, often appearing in Trust nursing strategies, proclaiming the search for new and more flexible ways of working; from the consideration given by Trusts to developing Band 4 posts; or more tangibly from the initiatives taken to develop the role, as with the Emergency Department Technician at London. But the main findings suggested that the HCA role rarely figured on the corporate or even the divisional agenda in prominent and proactive ways.

This situation was apparent partly in the fact that any consideration of the HCA role at corporate level was usually within the context of a skill mix review. While such reviews could be linked to broader, forward looking Trust goals related to the (more) even and patient-sensitive distribution of staff resources and improvements in care quality, they were more typically guided by more pressing issues associated with cost efficiency. This was reflected not least in the fact that the most recent, thorough skill mix review, accompanied by a workforce reduction programme, had been completed in Midlands, the Trust facing the most pressing financial pressures. It was also evident in the compression of the HCA workforce into Band 2, a pattern hardly suggestive of a careful consideration of how Band 2 and Band 3 roles might be used to deliver care. Indeed this compression within Band 2 was perhaps a further indicator of the HCA role being driven by cost concerns. It was a finding reinforced by the disordered alignment of pay band, qualification, and tasks across the Trusts.

This cost-efficient approach to the HCA workforce might well have been driven by the ease with which Band 2 HCAs could be recruited across Trusts: as a ready source of cheap labour, there was little incentive for Trusts to consider more imaginative ways of attracting individuals to the role or innovating on its use. However, this approach also reflects a more general weakness in workforce planning across Trusts: the HCA role was not alone in being considered in an ad hoc and opportunistic way—this characterized the broader approach to workforce issues. There was little evidence of what might be labelled a strategic HR management approach in Trusts, linking the development of work roles and other HR practices to corporate goals. The HR agenda at this level had rather been narrowed and driven by compliance: at board and executive level much HR interest and activity revolved around the monitoring of selective workforce targets, for instance, related to the level of staff absence, turnover, the use of agency staff, and completion of PDRs.

Backgrounds

Demand for HCAs, crudely driven by skill mix ratios, was formulated in broadly drawn job descriptions and founded upon low entry requirements, loosely interpreted by those recruiting at ward level. A plentiful supply of applicants, albeit of uneven quality, was elicited in this way. The result was HCA workforces across the four case study Trusts which shared a number of qualities related to their personal features, career histories, motivation, working and employment patterns. In short, an unregulated care support role positioned within the secondary healthcare sector of the NHS attracted those with similar background characteristics regardless of Trust or location.

In terms of shared personal features, HCAs tended to be middle-aged women with children and partners, well embedded in the local community. Moreover they were distinguished from nurses in being much less likely to have an ethnic background and more likely to have roots in the local community. Career histories were typically diverse, with work experience in a range of sectors— heath, social care, education, retail, and manufacturing—as well as in a non-paid domestic setting. Gateways into the HCA role were, however, limited: for many HCAs the last job before assuming their role was in the social care or healthcare sector.

Individual engagement with the HCA role was also underpinned by a limited number of shared narratives rationalizing this career choice: re-connecting to a disrupted nurse career; building on a personal care experience; and becoming a registered nurse. The survey data suggested that ambition to become a nurse was a particularly strong narrative amongst prospective HCAs.

The background of HCAs did, however, vary, especially by Trust, in part reflecting local labour conditions, and the associated industrial structure of the catchment area, but also a consequence of differences in corporate cultures, policies, and practices. For example, the Trust located in the most ethnically diverse area had a significantly higher proportion of HCAs with a BME background than other Trusts; in addition, some Trusts had been better able than others to recruit HCAs deeply embedded in the community. It was apparent that the tightness of the labour market created some HCA recruitment difficulties on one site in one Trust, while the looseness of that market provided greater choice in the selection of candidates in another Trust, reflected in the higher proportion of HCAs with a social care background. Moreover, the significantly higher HCA union density in one Trust likely reflected a more entrenched tradition of trade union membership; with the regularization of shift working in another Trust directly related to the introduction of an e-rostering system.

The shape of the HCA role

In exploring the shape of the HCA role, consideration was given to the often overlooked question of who the HCA is actually assisting or supporting. There were different emphases placed by different actors on whether the HCA supported the nurse, the team, or the patient: the nurse was more likely to view the HCA as a nurse support, the ward manager as a team support, and the HCA as a patient support. These differences of emphases spilled over into perceptions of the 'good' HCA: thus, while 'caring' was seen by all actors as the most important characteristic, HCAs were more inclined to stress the importance of patience and empathy with the patient, while nurses stressed the significance of HCA initiative and ward managers the value of the HCA as co-worker.

Central to unpacking the shape of the HCA role, however, were attempts to characterize and then explain the various forms assumed by it. The characterization of the HCA role revolved around notions of core and extension. Public policy developments appeared to have encouraged the role to move away from traditional nurse auxiliary activities, typically revolving around routine ward maintenance tasks. The more recent focus was on direct and indirect patient care, overlapping and perhaps even replacing the registered nurse as the lead care provider, with further scope to take on more technical and specialist tasks.

Our observation data provided some support for these developments, suggesting that HCAs were spending much more of their time on the provision of direct and indirect care than nurses. At the same time, it was noted that a more refined shaping of the role was linked to four sets of factors: the Trust, the division, the ward, and the individual.

The survey data provided a much sharper picture of the different forms assumed by the HCA role. Five HCA types were distinguished, varying in the diversity and complexity of tasks performed:

- the Bedside Technician (medium complexity/medium diversity);
- the Ancillary (low complexity/low diversity);
- the Citizen (medium complexity/high diversity);
- the All Rounder (high complexity/high diversity);
- the Expert (high complexity/low diversity).

With the Ancillary seen to constitute the remnants of the traditional nursing auxiliary, the Bedside Technician emerged as the new standard model. The Bedside Technician remained distinct from the registered nurse in not carrying out the full array of technical tasks, but as the new standard model, it was a role which undertook routine technical tasks such as BMs and observations, as well as regular direct and indirect care work. The All Rounder and the Expert HCAs were noteworthy in scoring high on complexity, indicative of some role extension, although the numbers in these roles were limited, suggesting some constraint on the scope for this extension.

The distribution of these HCA role types was related to the Trust, with a significant proportion of HCAs in two hospitals found to be Bedside Technicians, while another had a relatively high proportion of Ancillary HCAs. Unpacking the reasons for these patterns was far from straightforward: in the latter case it might have been related to the collapse of NVQ accreditation creating problems in signalling advanced skills, but elsewhere latent elements in terms of path-dependent values, practices, and routines might well have been at work.

Other patterns were more transparent. The influence of structure was revealed in the greater concentration of the Bedside Technician in medical than in the surgical wards: the higher dependency and need for direct care of patients on these wards lending some plausibility to this finding. Clinical area was also important in accounting for the emergence of the Expert and the Citizen; while these types were not linked to broad clinical division, the make-up of these types was found to be heavily concentrated in certain areas. The exercise of agency was more apparent in the case of the All Rounder. Breaking through structural constraints was not easy: there were few All Rounders. However, the dispersion of those in this role across many clinical areas, allied to the fact that they were not performing in line with others on their ward, and the link between this type and personal aspirations suggested that the All Rounder was very much the product of individual job crafting.

Consequences

For each of the main actors with a stake in the HCA role—the post holders themselves, the nurses, and the patients—it was originally suggested that outcomes might plausibly assume a positive or negative form or some uneasy combination of the two. Indeed Table 10.1 summarizing the outcomes for the respective stakeholders, indicates that this latter, hybrid outcome was most in evidence. Across the three stakeholders there was often a disconnect between the qualitative and quantitative data on outcomes: in general, the qualitative material supported a positive scenario, while the quantitative findings typically presented a more qualified picture. It remains open to some debate as to why this was the case. The specific methods used might have encouraged particular responses: for example, a facilitated focus group might well have been more conducive to producing a positive patient view of the HCA than a questionnaire received largely unsolicited and completed by the respondent alone. On the other hand, this disconnect may well reflect a genuine ambiguity amongst actors about the consequences of the HCA role. In the case of nurses, for example, this ambiguity seems highly plausible: a reflection of contradictory elements within the nurse professionalization project. Similarly in the case of the patient, different views might well reflect the selective recollection of different types of interaction with the HCA.

HCA outcomes

For the HCAs, alone of the three actors, it was the qualitative data which gave a slightly stronger hint of negative outcomes than the quantitative.

Table 10.1 Stakeholder consequences

Stakeholder	Positive	Negative
HCAs	New opportunities:	Added work:
	• Job satisfaction	• Thwarted nurse aspirations
	• Intention to stay	• Effort–reward misalignment
	• Mainly in-role development	• Band 2 workforce
	• Few dislikes	• No voice
	• Convenient job	• Patchy appraisals
		• Limited bespoke training
Nurses	New support:	Added burdens:
	• HCA as relief	• Uncertain accountability
	• HCA as mentor	• Encroachment of job territory
	• HCA as partners	• Contingent relationship
	• HCA as extra eyes	• Qualified gains
Patients	New access:	Added uncertainty:
	• HCA as closer	• Co-production contested
	• HCA as less daunting	• Preference for nurses
	• HCA as more empathetic	
	• HCA with better caring behaviours	

The interview material suggested that the management of HCAs was problematic in a number of respects. The collective voice of the HCA was fragile: there was an absence of safe, Trust spaces or opportunities for HCAs to aggregate and express shared interests, while workplace trade union organization remained weak. Moreover, the misalignment of task, pay banding, and NVQ qualification, driven by the concentration of the HCA workforce in Band 2, had distorted the effort–reward bargain for some, especially those with an NVQ3, and others, in Band 2 performing extended roles. Indeed, this misalignment begged questions about how 'fairly' HCAs were being treated by their Trusts.

Selective HCAs also raised some concerns about their role and their treatment—a lack of respect and of recognition, a sense that they were sometimes 'dumped-on'. More generally, the HCA role emerged as emotionally intense, although the impact of such intensity on the quality of working life was heavily contingent on the circumstances of the emotional experience and the individual HCA's coping strategy. Indeed, depending on interpretive coping responses from HCAs, emotional labour could emerge as contributing considerably to job enrichment.

Certainly in interview, many of the HCAs did stress the enjoyment they gained from their work, the source of such enjoyment often lying in the contact with patients. This positive view of their role was confirmed in the survey data, which revealed high HCA job satisfaction across the Trusts, and few signs of intention to leave. These data also suggested that while a majority of post holders in each Trust saw themselves as remaining and developing in the HCA role, a considerable minority continued to hold out the hope of becoming a registered nurse. The HCA role did not appear to 'squeeze out' this ambition, a number of HCAs retaining it for many years. An individual adherence to this ambition might be viewed with some poignancy given the major institutional and personal barriers which HCAs faced in moving on to nurse training.

Nurse outcomes

The qualitative data indicated that nurses viewed HCAs in an extremely positive way across all Trusts: in interview, nurses stressed the value of the HCA contribution to the ward team, often suggesting that the ward could not function without them. It was a picture confirmed in observation. This revealed few workplace problems between HCA and nurses, and workplace routines which reflected smooth and cooperative forms of working. Certainly nurses perceived some tensions: nurses were 'niggled' by what they felt were misconceptions amongst some HCAs about their laziness; a 'them' and 'us' divide was occasionally noted which could reflect and spill over into the odd dispute about role boundaries. The most tangible nurse concern, however, related to accountability. There was some nervousness around nurse responsibility for the HCA, not least in the context of the vagaries around Trust policies on the delegation of tasks to HCAs and around the absence of statutory regulation of the role. At the same time, it was clear from the nurse perspective that the HCA was valued by the nurse not only as a relief but as a mentor, an 'extra pair of eyes' and a partner.

The nurse survey data presented a more nuanced picture. In general, nurses were more grudging in the value they placed on the HCA as a relief, and especially as mentor and an 'extra pair of eyes'. There were striking differences in nurse and HCA views on who performed certain routine direct and indirect care tasks: whilst HCAs felt that they mainly performed these tasks, nurses resolutely adhered to the view that they continued to deliver them.

Patient outcomes

The qualitative data from all stakeholders provided strong support for the positive scenario of the HCA as patient friend and confidant. Certainly, there were suggestions that patients had difficulty distinguishing HCAs from other members of the ward team, but there was a strong consensus that HCAs developed a closer relationship with patients than nurses, a relationship patients often felt more comfortable with. Views on the reasons for this distinctive relationship varied. HCAs spent more time with patients than nurses, often through the provision of personal care. For some, there was nothing intrinsic to the HCA role which allowed them to get closer to the patient; nurses with the same time on their hand would have been able to get just as close. Others felt that patients did find it easier to relate to those who carried out a lower level support role, and to the kind of people who performed it. This was a view which strongly emerged from the patients themselves, as apparent in the focus group discussions.

The survey data again presented a more complex picture. There was evidence to suggest that HCAs contributed in a distinctive way to patient care: it was apparent from these data that HCAs across all Trusts found it easier to deal with certain types of difficult patients and situations than nurses. However nurses were again more reluctant to stress the co-producing value of the HCAs than they had been in interview: when it came to specifying a number of ways in which HCAs and nurses might be more sensitive to patient needs and better able to develop a close relationship with them, in all Trusts nurses continued to score their performance highly, particularly relative to the HCAs. In short the nurse views on the capacity of HCAs to get closer to patients, was not mirrored in the nurse survey results.

Surveyed patients also presented a more qualified view of their relations with HCAs. A noteworthy majority of patients claimed to be able to distinguish between HCAs and nurses. This proportion did vary by Trust, suggesting the importance of local practice, although the main source of identification across all hospitals remained the uniform. Despite suggestions in the focus groups of a close relationship with HCAs, patients indicated in the survey that they preferred to deal with nurses than HCAs, particularly on questions related to their condition. Equally significant was the finding that across all Trusts those patients who could distinguish between HCAs and nurses had a better care experience. Our qualitative data indicated that this was a highly plausible finding: for example, knowing who to approach with a question or a form of care is likely to reduce frustration. It is also a finding which has significant policy implications. The next section of this chapter returns to public policy and, in particular, the extent to which the findings presented in this book support those policy assumptions related to the HCA role.

Public policy goals and assumptions

The initial rationale for this project was the growing importance attached by policymakers to the support worker role in secondary healthcare against the backdrop of public services reform and modernization. Articulated with varying degrees of explicitness, and not without a degree of ambiguity, the role was seen as a vehicle for pursuing a number of policy goals: thus, the HCA was seen as a relief, substitute, apprentice, and a co-producer. In addition we imputed a degree of strategic intent into the pursuit of these goals: any meaningful articulation of such aims might be seen as requiring at the very least some forward planning at senior management levels within Trusts. This section re-visits these policy intentions, and, in particular, reviews the support provided by our study for the assumptions which informed them. Table 10.2 summarizes the picture presented by the research. It can be seen that, in general, the research: casts considerable doubt on the adoption of strategic approaches toward the HCA role; provides strong support for the use of the HCA as relief; and presents mixed evidence on the role's use as a substitute, co-producer, and an apprentice. Each of these goals is now considered in more detail.

Table 10.2 Public policy goals

Purpose	Support	Opposition
Strategic approach		Little consideration at senior levels
		Poorly developed Trust wide systems
Relief	Extension to direct care	
Substitution	Routine technical tasks performed	Cost-driven skill mix reviews
		Limited attention to band mix
		Patient preferences (?)
		An exploitative arrangement (?)
Apprentice	High HCA aspirations	HCA barriers to training
		Poorly developed Trust workforce planning
		Limited training opportunities
Co-producer	HCAs deal with the difficult patients	Contested nurse/HCA views
	HCAs closer to patients	Patient preferences (?)

A strategic resource?

Drawing on a strong definition of 'the strategic' as a forward-looking approach which explicitly relates policy and practice to medium- and longer-term organizational objectives, it is difficult to conclude that Trusts viewed and used HCAs in a strategic manner. In general, Trusts were driven by pressing targets linked to patient access, finance, and other outcome measures, which senior managers were unable in any considered way to relate to workforce reform or planning, and certainly not to the support worker role. This was, for example, reflected in the concentration of HCAs in Band 2 and in the disordered relationship between pay band, qualification, and tasks performed. This is, however, a picture which needs to be qualified in a number of ways

- The scope to develop the support role in our clinical areas—general medical and surgical—might have been less obvious than in other, more specialist clinical areas. In some Trusts there were initiatives, but they tended to be in such areas as emergency care and theatres.

- There were differences in Trust approaches to managing HCAs, apparent in contrasting policy and practice. For example, the level of NVQ accreditation varied markedly; some Trusts were more successful than others in aligning Band 3s with NVQ 3s; while there was some unevenness between Trusts in how easy it was for patients to identify HCAs. These are variations which imply an opportunity for Trusts to address the HCA role in a more considered way: this might not be a 'grand strategy' as defined earlier, but clearly there was scope for senior management to plan and more explicitly acknowledge the HCA's contribution to patient care. Most obviously, it is clear from our research that a Trust-wide approach which facilitated patient identification of HCAs would likely improve patient perceptions of their care experience.

- Closely related, the research revealed different patterns in the distribution of various types of HCA between Trusts. Uncovering the reasons for these differences was not easy; they may well lay in 'deep' and path-dependent structures, systems and values. Nonetheless, in revealing these differences, our research encourages Trusts more explicitly to build upon the forms assumed by the HCA role and their particular contribution to patient care.

A relief?

The research provided some support for the development of the HCA role as a relief for nurses, taking some of the more 'routine' tasks from them and freeing them up to concentrate on more technical, specialist clinical tasks. Both the qualitative and quantitative data suggested that the HCA is the primary provider of direct and indirect care, nurses being distinguished from the standard HCA in carrying out a greater range of more complex tasks. This had bred some discontent amongst HCAs, occasionally viewing themselves as the 'work horses' of the ward and as being 'dumped on'. But such concerns did not feed through to job satisfaction, which remained high. Indeed in relieving nurses of direct care tasks, HCAs were often brought into close contact with patients, an aspect of the role they found particularly rewarding. Moreover, nurses also seemed to greatly value the HCA in helping in these respects, although there was some residual nurse ambiguity about the implications of these developments for their claims to the provision of holistic care.

A substitute?

A more qualified picture emerges as to whether and how effectively the HCA was being used as a substitute for the nurse. It was striking that the new standard HCA, the Bedside Technician, was not only undertaking direct and indirect care tasks but also performing routine technical tasks such as observations and BMs. In short, the HCA had not only relieved nurses of routine direct care tasks but was now also a partner in the delivery of some lower-level technical ones. This might be viewed as falling within the HCA's role as a relief, but equally it could be argued that by taking on such tasks, HCAs were beginning to encroach on some traditional core registered nurse tasks. Certainly such low-level technical tasks might be seen to constitute the borders of the professional role, which HCAs had now colonized.

Skill mix reviews were being undertaken in a number of Trusts, and had in certain instances led to some reconfiguration of grades rather than a fundamental rebalancing of registered and unregistered staff, which might crudely be viewed as dilution. It might well be argued that in taking on routine technical tasks on a partnership basis with nurses, HCAs were increasingly substituting for nurses in these spheres of activity. Moreover, the boundaries between the HCA and nurse were fairly broadly drawn, with the limits of the HCA role lying in the exclusive nurse dispensation of medication and patient assessment, allowing considerable scope for HCA role extension. However, our data suggested that while some HCAs were performing more extended roles, the number should not be overstated: the HCA All Rounder and the Expert, those role types at the high complexity end of the scale, were fairly limited in numbers.

Caution about the claims that HCAs were being used as substitutes in this sense should not, however, detract from the misalignment between pay band, formal qualification, and tasks performed. The concentration of the HCA workforce in Band 2 had resulted in a distortion in the effort–reward bargain for some, particularly those with advanced capabilities, typically but not invariably signalled by NVQ 3. It was where the HCA was in Band 2, performing an extended role with or without an NVQ 3, that the issue of 'fairness' and notions of 'cheap labour' most obviously emerged. Indeed, it is in this respect that a creeping, almost 'subterranean', form of substitution might be identified.

An apprentice?

The research provided considerable support for the HCA as an apprentice, both in terms of the individual post holder developing within the role to become a 'high performing HCA' and as a potential source for future registered nurses. Most HCAs saw their future as HCAs, with many of these keen to develop within the role. The uneven approach to training within Trusts, the patchiness of completion of PDRs and the general absence of workplace planning at any level, raised some doubt about the efficiency and effectiveness with which Trusts were addressing these enthusiastic HCAs keen to develop within the role.

More striking was the significant stock of HCAs willing to become registered nurses. This was often a rationale for becoming an HCA, with many individuals holding nurse aspirations on taking up the role. It was a remarkably durable aspiration, which only faded after many years in the HCA role. Indeed it was the very durability of this aspiration, allied to continuing and significant barriers faced by HCAs in becoming registered nurses, which suggests the need for a more considered approach to this issue amongst policymakers at different levels. There are grounds for drawing upon the enthusiasm of HCAs who wish to become a nurse, and supporting it by reducing the barriers they face in developing their careers. However, given these barriers, such an approach needs to be balanced by a shaping of HCA expectations: from the outset, HCAs need to be aware of and sensitive to the difficulties faced in achieving nurse status.

A co-producer?

The research lent strong support to the suggestion that HCAs brought distinctive capabilities to the provision of healthcare. Indeed, our research might be seen as a counter to the deluge of recent concern, particularly from the professional nurse establishment that HCAs represented a threat to care standards and an undesirable source of risk. This distinctive contribution was seen to take a number of forms.

- HCAs did have different backgrounds to nurses, most significantly being more deeply rooted in the local community. They also had a breadth and richness of work experience which suggested they brought with them to the role a range of tacit skills and capabilities.

- Much of the evidence suggested that HCAs were able to develop a closer relationship with patients than nurses, a closeness which patients themselves put down to being able to relate more easily to HCAs than nurses.

- There was also firm data to indicate that HCAs 'added value' by more easily being able to deal with certain types of difficult patient than nurses. Indeed HCAs found it easier to deal with verbally abusive patients and deeply upset patients than nurses.

The value of HCAs as co-producers in these terms should not obscure the apparent preference of patients to deal with nurses rather than HCAs on certain issues. However, this only strengthens the suggestion that the quality of care is likely to be improved if patients are more clearly informed about the differences between the roles of respective ward team members.

Future developments

In this final section of the book attention turns to future developments. These developments relate both to the HCA role and to how it might be further studied. Clearly these areas of future interest overlap: how the role evolves will influence the nature and focus of a forward-looking research agenda. The evolution of the role is likely to be heavily contingent on broader developments, the most important being whether plans to regulate it are taken forward. Policy developments in this respect remain ongoing and fluid. At the time of writing, the government has announced its intention to introduce a voluntary register for support workers in health and social care, along with certain minimum training standards and a Code of Conduct, with the Council for Healthcare Regulatory Excellence responsible for managing and overseeing the process. There are still a range of questions that need to be addressed in seeking to implement a form of regulation along these lines:

- Coverage: whether HCAs as a generic group will be covered by this regulation, or whether it will apply more selectively to, say, APs at Band 4.

- Enforcement: whether or not voluntary registration will be tied to the Code of Conduct and the achievement of minimum training standards, and if so how those who fail to meet or breach these requirements, or those deciding not to sign on to the register, will be handled or viewed by Trusts and others.

- Cost: whether the costs of this form of regulation, including those costs associated with training and registration, will be borne by the Trust and or by the individual employee.

Notwithstanding the resolution of these residual uncertainties, the findings from our study suggest that this, and indeed most, forms of regulation are likely to impact in various ways upon on the HCA role. They are likely to influence Trust views on and use of the HCA role: the additional costs associated with regulation might encourage a review of its value for money, although tighter regulation might also prompt greater use of the role with more assurance on clinical governance and quality standard issues. Such regulation might also impact on individual decisions to take up the role or remain within it: (potential) post holders might be unable to meet the costs associated with registration and training, and/or be intimidated by the prospect of needing to acquire higher accredited qualifications.

Setting aside the uncertainties associated with the development of new forms of regulation, it is still possible to speculate as to the future development of the HCA role and the research issues this might generate. There is scope for the HCA role at Bands 1–4 to develop along three main lines: management of the role; creation of new work roles; and role extension.

Management of the role

We have seen that in important respects the management of the HCA role has been weak and underdeveloped. As the service delivery and financial pressures on Trusts intensify, consideration might be given to the better management of HCAs. This would involve addressing how HCA are: recruited, trained, supervised, appraised, rewarded, and involved.

New work roles

A new work role is one which reconfigures the bundling of task and responsibilities in a novel way. We have seen that much public policy has been focused on encouraging the development of such roles as a means of dealing more efficiently and effectively with services needs, in particular breaking down some of the occupational barriers to the delivery of flexible, patient-centred services.

Extended roles

It has been noted that the role of the HCAs has been progressively extended over the years, with the potential for further development in this respect. Role extension might again be driven by the search for new, more efficient and effective forms of service delivery, but it constitutes a less radical, more incremental approach to job redesign than the creation of new roles. Such role extension is founded on the HCA retaining an established core to their role, but taking on some additional tasks and responsibilities.

The identification of these three lines of potential development open up a number of research questions for future consideration. Most obviously, these are questions about whether, how and why Trusts are seeking to develop the HCA role along these lines. More specifically:

- Are certain of these lines of development more common than others, and if so, does this suggest that some are 'easier' to take forward, or perhaps more pressing?

- Are certain Trusts more efficient and effective in developing these initiatives than others, implying that organizational architecture plays some part in facilitating or inhibiting change?

- Are certain lines of development to be found in particular clinical areas, a signal that some service areas are more open or amenable to change, or again that this particular change is more pressing in specific areas?

- Are certain regions of the country more likely to develop the HCA role along these lines, perhaps a legacy of the different levels of support provided by SHAs for various initiatives?

Those questions which focus on the potentially uneven development and management of the HCA role *between* Trusts assume particular interest: after all our main unit of analysis has been the Trust and as the employer, the Trust is likely to be responsible for taking forward (or not) any initiative. It is an intriguing issue as to why some Trusts are willing and able to take forward the HCA role along some or all three of the lines distinguished, while others are not. Addressing this issue suggests a need to turn inwards and explore Trust architecture or infrastructure. External factors might well retain their importance. For example, certain SHAs, particularly the North West, and to a lesser extent the East of England, pursued the development of new roles at the Band 4 AP level with particular alacrity, providing resource to Trusts to support them in this respect. However, the main locus of interest remains the Trust: whether its organizational set-up facilitates or inhibits change along any or all of the three lines distinguished.

This is not the place to unpack the notion of 'organizational architecture', beyond a general reference to its focus on culture, leadership and management styles, work and employment systems. Nonetheless, it is worth briefly reviewing contemporary movements along the three lines distinguished in developing the HCA role, and any available evidence on the emergence of organization infrastructure to support such movement. Further research work on the HCA role, covering Bands 1–4, has been undertaken since the completion of the study reported in this book. This section draws upon this work—mainly interviews and workshops with various actors at Trust and regional level

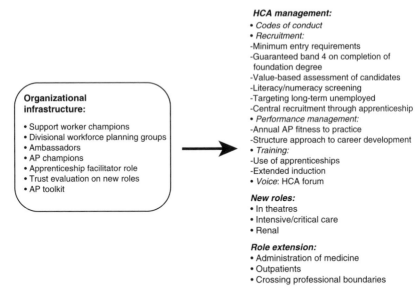

Organizational infrastructure:

- Support worker champions
- Divisional workforce planning groups
- Ambassadors
- AP champions
- Apprenticeship facilitator role
- Trust evaluation on new roles
- AP toolkit

HCA management:
- *Codes of conduct*
- *Recruitment:*
-Minimum entry requirements
-Guaranteed band 4 on completion of foundation degree
-Value-based assessment of candidates
-Literacy/numeracy screening
-Targeting long-term unemployed
-Central recruitment through apprenticeship
- *Performance management:*
-Annual AP fitness to practice
-Structure approach to career development
- *Training:*
-Use of apprenticeships
-Extended induction
- *Voice*: HCA forum

New roles:
- In theatres
- Intensive/critical care
- Renal

Role extension:
- Administration of medicine
- Outpatients
- Crossing professional boundaries

Figure 10.1 Overview of contemporary developments.

designed to explore key issues associated with the role and how it is being developed.

Figure 10.1 provides an overview of recent developments. In terms of organizational infrastructure, it appears from the figure that some Trusts are setting up working groups to explore the management and use of HCAs. Most striking, however, is the emergence of a number of specialist roles within Trusts as advocates or supports for taking forward the HCA role: 'champions' and 'ambassadors'. These are perhaps signs of slightly more strategic orientation amongst some Trusts to the nurse support role.

As for the three lines of development, most activity is apparent in attempts to 'improve' the management of the HCA, with particular effort put into tightening recruitment to these roles. Such tightening is reflected in the introduction of literacy and numeracy tests to screen candidates and in the use of values-based recruitment to more intensively assess the suitability of applicants for the role. Closely related, Trusts have been using the Qualifications and Credit Framework (QCF) training model, replacing NVQs, and apprenticeships to structure entry into and development within the HCA role: for instance, in some Trusts confirmation to the post is only granted once the appropriate qualifications are acquired, with a time limit for their achievement. Indeed a few Trusts are beginning to use Band 1 as a training grade. Developments along the other two lines—new roles and role extension—have been more uneven, perhaps unsurprising given the clinical governance issues raised in these cases. Low-risk areas, like outpatient clinics, provide opportunities for HCAs to extend their roles, but there are also instances of role development in high-risk areas, such as intensive care, and in relation to higher-risk procedures such as the administration of medication.

Against the backdrop of these specific moves, there remains considerable debate about the scope for developing the HCA role, how this might be taken forward, and what form it might take. This debate comprises a number of tensions or competing views, with a Trust's approach to the HCA role often depending on where it sits in relation to such matters. These structural tensions are each summarized in turn.

- *The value of apprenticeships and the QCF:* for some Trusts the use of apprenticeships and the QCF provides a more viable means of training and accrediting HCAs than the old NVQ system. The QCF, in particular, is seen as a more flexible, incremental approach to the development of HCAs. However, there are also suggestions that apprenticeships create rigidities, tying HCAs into lengthy periods of training and inhibiting the speedy take-up of the full role.

- *Sources of funding:* there is uncertainty about future sources of funding for new role development, especially at AP level. At the same time, concerns have been raised about Trust reliance of external funding for these purposes. There might well be a temptation for Trusts to chase available money for development of particular roles, without careful consideration of whether the roles in question are needed

- *Career progression and cost constraints:* in the current financial environment, an emphasis on developing careers from Bands 2–4 has to confront the cost pressures which suggest a 'need' to contain support workers in Band 2. In short, calls to develop HCAs across the Band 2–4 spectrum sit uneasily with the likely downward pressure on labour costs.

- *Bottom up or top down role development:* there is a considerable difference in emphasis between Trusts seeking to develop the HCA workforce through the initial development of APs at Band 4 and those more concerned with ensuring that those in the lower bands are comfortable and competent in their roles.

- *Band focus:* partly related, Trusts differ in their band focus. For some, there is a concern to 'sweat' Band 2s further, and before even considering the development of Band 4 roles. For others, there is a broader interest in 'sorting out' Bands 2 and 3s; that is, in untangling their respective tasks and responsibilities. There are other instances where Bands 2 and 4, in particular, are the key bands, whilst in yet others cases Band 3 rather than 4 is the pivotal role.

• *Assistant practitioner versus Band 5:* views differ on the value for money associated with AP roles, particularly relative to the Band 5 registered nurse. Although the direct labour costs associated with the APs are lower, these remain unregistered roles, with some Trusts still therefore seeing the registered nurse at Band 5 as a more useful and valuable resource. There are concerns about the quality of the evidence base on the use of APs, which adds to these doubts about the role's value for money.

• *Grow your own:* for some, the Band 4 AP role is seen as an important source of future registered nurses. Indeed, taking the individual from Band 2 through Band 4 to nurse status at Band 5 is regarded by some Trusts as a viable career route. Other Trusts are more cautious about using Band 4s as a feeder into registered nursing, arguing that retaining a stable group of APs is the surest means of supporting moves to allow registered nurses to return to the provision of more direct patient care.

From the debates and tensions swirling around the HCA role, it is clear that future development remains uncertain. A role whose 'time has come' is not yet clear quite what this 'coming of age' might in practice mean or entail. Recognizing the renewed importance of HCAs to their performance and well-being in the current climate, Trusts are scampering around in search of a more coherent and considered approach to the HCA role. In this book we have sought to provide a firmer basis for these deliberations: an appreciation of those who take up the role—the kinds of people they are, the sorts of pressures they face, and the aspirations they hold; an understanding of what they do—the varied forms the role takes, the differences behind the shared job title; and an appreciation of how the role impacts—on those who undertake it, on those who work alongside it, and on those cared for by it. The HCA role is no longer one policymakers and practitioners at national, regional, and Trust level can leave behind the scenes to develop unevenly, randomly, and incrementally. It is hoped that this book, in providing the most detailed and comprehensive evidence base of the role to date, will contribute to these future deliberations.

References

Abbott A. *The system of Professions: An Essay on the Division of Expert Labour*. Chicago, IL: University of Chicago Press; 1988.

Allen D. *The Changing Shape of Nurse Practice: The Role of Nurses in the Hospital Division of Labour*. London: Routledge; 2001.

Australian Nursing Federation. *A snapshot of nursing in Australia. Fact Sheet 2*. Canberra: ANF; 2011.

Bach S, Kessler I. *The Modernisation of the Public Services and Employee Relations*. London: Palgrave Macmillan; 2011.

Bach S, Kessler I, Heron P. Role redesign in a modernised NHS: The case of HCAs. *Human Resource Management Journal* 2008; 58(2): 171–87.

Barley S, Kunda G. Bringing work back in. *Organizational Science* 2001; 12(1): 76–95.

BBC. Nurses cannot be too posh to wash. *BBC* [Online] 10 May 2004; Available at: http://news.bbc.co.uk/1/hi/health/3701855.stm [Accessed 12 December 2011].

Bolton S. *Emotion Management in the Workplace*. Basingstoke: Palgrave; 2005.

Bosley S, Dale J. Healthcare assistants in general practice: practical and conceptual issues of skill mix change. *British Journal of General Practice* 2008; 58: 118–24.

Brennan G, McSherry R. Exploring the transition and professional socialisation from health care assistant to student nurse. *Nurse Education in Practice* 2007; 7(4): 206–14.

Briggs A. *Report of the Committee on Nursing*. London: HMSO; 1972.

Brown A, Jones K. *Modernising Nursing Careers, Advanced and Specialist Nursing Practice— A Scoping Report*. London: NHS London; 2011.

Buchan J. *Nurse Workforce Planning in the UK: A Report for the RCN*. London: RCN; 2007.

Buchan J, Seccombe I. *Behind the headlines*. London: RCN; 2002.

Camano-Puig R. *Professionalisation of nursing in England and Spain: A comparative study*. Helsinki: Laurea Publications; 2005.

Care Quality Commission. *Dignity and Nutrition Inspection Programme National Overview*. Newcastle Upon Tyne: CQC; 2011.

Carr-Hill R, Dixon P, Gibbs I, Griffiths M, Higgins M, McMaughan D, Wright K. *Skill mix and effectiveness of nursing care*. York: Centre for Health Economics, University of York; 1992.

Chang A. Perceived functions and usefulness of health service support workers. *Journal of Advanced Nursing* 1995; 21: 64–74.

Chang A, Lam L. Can HCAs replace student nurses? *Journal of Advanced Nursing* 1998; 27(2): 399–405.

Cox A, Grimshaw D, Carroll M, McBride A. Reshaping internal labour markets in the NHS: New Prospect for pay and training for lower skilled serve workers? *Human Resource Management Journal* 2008; 18(4): 347–65.

Daly T, Szebehely M. Unheard voices, unmapped terrain: care work in long-term residential care for older people in Canada and Sweden. *International Journal of Social Welfare* 2011; DOI: 10.1111/j.1468–2397.2011.00806.x.

Daykin N, Clarke B. 'They'll still get bodily care'. Discourses of care and relationships between nurses and HCAs in the NHS. *Sociology of Health and Illness* 2000; 22(3): 349–63.

Delamaire M, Lafortune G. *Nurses in Advanced Roles: A Description and Evaluation of Experiences in 12 Developed Countries.* OECD Health Working Papers No.54. Paris: OECD Publishing; 2010.

Department of Health. *Working together, learning together: a framework for lifelong learning for the NHS.* London: HMSO; 2001.

Department of Health. *Delivering the HR in the NHS plan.* London: HMSO; 2003a.

Department of Health. *Speech by Sarah Mullally, Chief Nursing Officer, Keynote Address CNO Conference.* Department of Health [Online] 2003b; Available at: http://webarchive.nationalarchives.gov.uk/20040209012729/http://doh.gov.uk/speeches/mullallycnoconferencenov03.htm [Accessed 12 December 2011].

Department of Health. *The Regulation of Health Care Staff in England and Wales.* London: HMSO; 2004.

Department of Health. *The regulation of the non-medical healthcare professions: A review by the Department of Health.* London: HMSO; 2006a.

Department of Health. *Modernising Nursing Careers: Setting the Direction.* London: HMSO; 2006b.

Department of Health. *Trust, Assurance and Safety: The regulation of Health Professionals in the 21st Century.* London: HMSO; 2007a.

Department of Health. *Towards a framework for post registration nursing careers.* London: HMSO; 2007b.

Department of Health. *Introduction to the Skills Escalator.* Department of Health [Online] 2007c; Available at: http://webarchive.nationalarchives.gov.uk/+/www.dh.gov.uk/en/Managingyourorganisation/Humanresourcesandtraining/Modelcareer/DH_4055527 [Accessed 12 December 2011].

Department of Health. *High Quality Care for Next Stage Review.* London: HMSO; 2008.

Department of Health. *Extending Professional and Occupational Regulation: The Report of the Working Group on Extending Professional Regulation.* London: HMSO; 2009a.

Department of Health. *High Quality Workforce.* London: HMSO; 2009b.

Department of Health. *Enabling Excellence: Autonomy and Accountability for Healthcare Workers, Social Workers and Social Care Workers.* London: HMSO; 2011.

Dovlo D. Using mid-level cadres as substitutes for internationally mobile health professionals in Africa. A desk review. *Human Resources for Health* 2004; 2(7): 1–12.

Dingwell R. Atrocity stories and professional relationships. *Sociology of Work and Occupations* 1977; 4: 317–96.

Doherty C. 'The Effect of Jurisdictional Change on the Professionalisation of Nursing.' London: Unpublished DPhil Thesis, King's College, London; 2007.

Elliot B, Skatun D, Farrar S, Napper M. *The impact of local labour factors on the organisation and delivery of health services.* Final report. London: NCCSDO; 2003.

ERHC. *Close to Home: An Inquiry into older people and human rights in home care.* Manchester: ERHC; 2011.

European Commission. *Study of Specialist Nurses in Europe.* MARKT/D/8031/2000. Brussels: European Commission; 2000.

Fineman S. *Emotion and Organisations*. London: Sage; 1993.

Ford P. The role of support workers in the department of diagnostic imaging: service managers' perspectives. *Radiography* 2004; 10: 259–67.

Francis R. *Independent Inquiry into care provided by Mid Staffordshire NHS Foundation Trust January 2005 - March 2009, Volumes 1 and 2*. London: HMSO; 2010.

Fullbrook S. Changing roles and titles: HCAs now deliver the care. *British Journal of Nursing* 2004; 13(14): 861.

Furaker C. Health care assistants' and mental attendants' daily tasks in acute hospital care. *Journal of Research in Nursing* 2008; 13(6): 542–53.

Gonzalez B, Barber, P. 'Planning for a well-skilled nursing and social care workforce in Europe. Case studies from Finland, Germany, Italy, Lithuania and Spain.' Prepared for Policy Dialogu; Venice, Italy; 11–12 May 2009.

Gottems LBD, Alves ED, Sena RR. Brazilian nursing and professionalisation at technical level: a retrospective analysis. *Rev Latino-am Enfermagem* 2007; 15(5): 1033–40.

Gould D, Carr G, Kelly D. Seconding healthcare assistants to a pre-registration nursing course. *Journal of Research in Nursing* 2006; 11(6): 561–72.

Gould R, Thompson D, Raquel B, Jenson J, Hasselman E, Young L. Redesigning the RN and NA roles. *Nursing Management* 1996; 27(2): 37–47.

Government of Canada. *Working in Canada Report. Occupation: Nurse Aides, Orderlies and Patient Service Associates (NOC 3413-C)*. Government of Canada Website 2011 [Online]; Available at: http://www.workingincanada.gc.ca/report-eng.do?noc=3413&action=search_occupation_confirm [Accessed 12 December 2011].

Grimshaw D. Changes in the skill mix and pay determination amongst the nursing workforce in the UK. *Work, Employment and Society* 1999; 13(2): 295–328.

Hancock C. Developing the role of the HCA. *Nursing Standard* 2006; 20(49): 35–51.

Hansard. *HC deb 24 Feb*. 1999: cc 364–71.

Hardie M, Hockey L. (eds.) *Nursing Auxiliaries in Health Care*. London: Croom Helm; 1978.

Hasson H, Arnetz JE. Nursing staff competence, work strain, stress and satisfaction in elderly care: a comparison of home-based care and nursing homes. *Journal of Clinical Nursing* 2008; 17(4): 468–81.

Healthcare Commission. *Acute Hospital Portfolio Review, Ward Staffing 2005*. London: Commission for Healthcare Audit and Inspection; 2005.

Healthcare Commission. *Investigation into outbreaks of Clostridium difficile at Maidstone and Tunbridge Wells NHS Trust*. London: Commission for Healthcare Audit and Inspection; 2007.

Hochschild A. *The Managed Heart*. Berkeley, CA: University of California Press; 1983.

Hogan J, Playle J. The utilisation of the healthcare assistant role in intensive care. *British Journal of Nursing* 2000; 9(12): 794–801.

Hongoro C, McPake B. How to bridge the gap in human resources for health. *Lancet* 2004; 364: 1451–6.

House of Commons Health Committee. *Workforce Planning: Fourth Report of Session 2006–07, Vol 1.HC 171–1*. London: HMSO; 2007.

HRSDC. *3413 Nurse Aides, Orderlies and Patient Service Associates*. Human Resources and Skills Development Canada Website 2006 [Online]; Available at: http://www5.hrsdc.

gc.ca/NOC/English/NOC/2006/Profile.aspx?val=3&val1=3413 [Accessed 12 December 2011].

Hughes EC. *The Sociological Eye*. London: Transaction; 1993.

Imison C, Buchan J, Xavier S. *NHS Workforce Planning: Limitations and Possibilities*. London: King's Fund; 2009.

Jack B, Brown J, Chapman T. Ward managers' perceptions of the role of HCAs. *British Journal of Nursing* 2004; 13(5): 270–5.

James N. Care = organisation + physical labour + emotional labour. *Sociology of Health and Illness* 1992; 14(4): 488–509.

Johnson M. Big fleas have little fleas—nurse professionalism and nursing auxiliaries. In: Hardie M, Hockey L. (eds) *Nursing Auxiliaries in Health Care*. London: Croom Helm; 1978, pp. 103–18.

Johnson M, Ormandy P, Long A, Hulme C. The role and accountability of senior health care support workers in ICUs. *Intensive and Critical Care Nursing* 2004; 20(3): 123–32.

Kalisch BJ, Liu Y. Comparison of nursing: China and the United States. *Nursing Economics* [Online] 2009; Sept–Oct; Available at: http://findarticles.com/p/articles/mi_m0FSW/is_5_27/ai_n39397730/?tag=content;col1 [Accessed 12 December 2011].

Keeney S, Hasson F, McKenna H. Health care assistants: the views of managers of health care agencies on training and employment. *Journal of Nursing Management* 2005; 13(1): 83–92.

Kessler I, Bach S, Heron P. 'The Role of the Public Service Support Workers.' Invited plenary session, a paper presented to Employment Research Unit Conference, Cardiff University; 2005.

Kessler I, Heron P, Dopson S. *The occupational management of service user emotions: support workers and hospital patients*. Unpublished paper (under review); 2011.

Kessler I, Heron P, Dopson S. Indeterminacy and the regulation of task allocation: the shape of support roles in healthcare. *British Journal of Industrial Relations* 2012a (forthcoming, DOI: 10.1111/j.1467-8543.2012.00892x).

Kessler I, Heron P, Dopson S. Opening the window: managing death in the workplace. *Human Relations* 2012b (forthcoming, DOI: 10.1177/0018726711430002).

King's Fund. *How much of the NHS budget is spent on workforce?* King's Fund [Online] 2010; Available at: http://www.kingsfund.org.uk/current_projects/general_election_2010/frequently_asked.html [Accessed 12 December 2011].

Knibb W, Smith P, Magnusson C, Bryan K. *The Contribution of Assistants to Nursing: Report for the RCN*. Guildford: University of Surrey; 2006.

Langlands A. *Gateways to the Professions Report*. London: DfES; 2005.

LPN Duties. *The duties of a licensed practical nurse (LPN)*. LPN Duties [Online] 2011; Available at: http://www.lpnduties.com/[Accessed 12 December 2011].

Maben J, Macleod Clark J. Project 2000 diplomates' perceptions of their experiences of transition from student to nurse. *Journal of Clinical Nursing* 1998; 7: 145–53.

Malhotra G. *Grow your own: creating the conditions for sustainable workforce development*. London: King's Fund; 2006.

Marsden D. *A Theory of Employment Systems*. Oxford: Oxford University Press; 1999.

Martin R. Politics and Industrial Relations. In: Ackers P, Wilkinson A. (Eds.) *Understanding Work and Employment*. Oxford: Oxford University Press; 2003, pp. 161–75.

May D, Smith L. Evaluation of the new ward housekeeper role in the UK NHS Trusts. *Facilities* 2003; 21(7/8): 168–74.

McCreight B. Perinatal grief and emotional labour: A study of nurses' experiences in gynea wards. *International Journal of Nursing Studies* 2005; 42(4): 439–48.

McKenna H, Hasson F, Keeney S. Patient safety of care: the role of HCAs. *Journal of Nursing Management* 2004; 12: 452–9.

McKenna H. Nursing Skills mix substitutions and quality of care: exploration of assumptions from the research literature. *Journal of Advanced Nursing* 1995; 21: 452–9.

McLaughlin FE, Barter M, Thomas SA, Rix G, Coulter M, Chadderton H. Perceptions of registered nurses working with assistive personnel in the UK and the US. *International Journal of Nursing Practice* 2000; 6: 46–57.

Malvarez S, Castrillon C. *Overview of the nursing workforce in Latin America, Issue paper 6. Human Resources Development Series No. 39*. Washington, DC: PAHO; 2005.

Meek R. Evaluation of the role of the healthcare assistant within a community mental health intensive care team. *Journal of Nursing Management* 1998; 6(1): 11–19.

Ministry of Health. *PROFAE: nursing workers professionalizing*. Brasillia: Ministry of Health; 2006.

Ministry of Health, Labour and Welfare. *Survey of Medical Institutions and Hospital Report*. Tokyo: MHLW; 2009.

Munjanja OK, Kibuka S, Dovlo D. *The nursing workforce in sub-Saharan Africa. Issue Paper 7*. Geneva: International Council of Nurses; 2005.

Neves E, Mauro M. Nursing in Brazil: trajectory, conquests and challenges. *Online Journal of Issues in Nursing* 2000; 6(1) [Online]; Available at: http://nursingworld.org/MainMenuCategories/ANAMarketplace/ANAPeriodicals/OJIN/TableofContents/Volume62001/No1Jan01/ArticlePreviousTopic/NursinginBrazil.aspx [Accessed 12 December 2011].

NHS Employers. *NHS Employers supports report on extending professional and occupational regulation*. NHS Employers [Online] 2009; Available at: http://www.nhsemployers.org/Aboutus/PressReleases/2009/Pages/extending-professional-and-occupational-regulation.aspx [Accessed 12 December 2011].

NHS Estates. *Housekeeping: A first guide to new, modern and dependable housekeeping services in the NHS*. London: HMSO; 2001.

NMC. *The Regulation of Health Care Support Workers: A Scoping Paper*. London: NMC; 2006.

Nursing Assistant Canada. Nursing Assistant Jobs. *Nursing Assistant Canada* 2011 [Online]; Available at: http://www.nursingassistant.ca/registered-nurse/nursing-assistant-jobs.html [Accessed 12 December 2011].

Nursing Council of New Zealand. *The New Zealand nursing workforce: A profile of nurse practitioners, registered nurses, nurse assistants and enrolled nurses*. Wellington: Nursing Council of New Zealand; 2010.

Nursing Times. Skill-mix and HCAs. *Nursing Times* [Online] 2007; 13 December; Available at: http://www.nursingtimes.net/whats-new-in-nursing/skill-mix-and-hcas/360917.article [Accessed 12 December 2011].

Nursing Times. Risks and benefits: Changing the nursing skill mix. *Nursing Times* [Online] 2009a; 22 September; Available at: http://www.nursingtimes.net/whats-new-in-nursing/acute-care/risks-and-benefits-changing-the-nursing-skill-mix/5006399.article [Accessed 12 December 2011].

Nursing Times. Hospitals to replace nursing posts with lower paid assistants. *Nursing Times* [Online] 2009b; 27 October; Available at: http://www.nursingtimes.net/whats-new-in-nursing/acute-care/hospitals-to-replace-nursing-posts-with-lower-paid-assistants/5007732.article [Accessed 12 December 2011].

Nursing Times. Regulation of HCA not a top priority for the NHS. *Nursing Times* 2011; 29 September; Available at: http://www.nursingtimes.net/nursing-practice-clinical-research/clinical-subjects/patient-experience/regulation-of-hca-not-a-top-priority-for-the-nhs/5035772.article [Accessed 12 December 2011].

Pan American Health Organization. *Health in the Americas, Volume II Colombia.* Washington, DC: PAHO; 2007.

Perry M, Carpenter I, Challis D, Hope K. Understanding the roles of registered general nurses and care assistants in UK nursing homes. *Journal of Advanced Nursing* 2003; 42(5): 497–505.

Philpin S. The impact of Project 2000 educational reforms on the occupational socialisation of nurses: An exploratory study. *Journal of Advanced Nursing* 1999; 29(6): 1326–31.

Power P, Dickey C, Ford A. Evaluating an RN/Co-worker model. *Journal of Nursing Administration* 1990; 20: 15–25.

RCN. *Maxi Nurses: Advanced and Specialist Nursing Roles.* London: RCN; 2005.

RCN. *Setting appropriate ward nurse staffing levels in NHS acute trusts: an exploration of the issues.* London: RCN Institute; 2006.

RCN. *RCN survey shows nurses spend more than a million hours a week on paperwork.* RCN [Online] 2008; Available at: http://www.rcn.org.uk/newsevents/news/article/uk/rcn_survey_shows_nurses_spend_more_than_a_million_hours_a_week_on_paperwork [Accessed 12 December 2011].

RCN. *NHS heading for crisis point as job losses mount.* RCN [Online] 2011a; Available at: http://www.rcn.org.uk/newsevents/news/article/uk/rcn_nhs_heading_for_crisis_point_as_job_losses_mount [Accessed 12 December 2011].

RCN. *Accountability and delegation: What you need to know.* RCN [Online] 2011b; Available at: http://www.rcn.org.uk/development/health_care_support_workers/accountability_and_delegation_film [Accessed 12 December 2011].

Reeve J. Nurses' attitudes towards healthcare assistants. *Nursing Times* 1994; 90: 43–6.

Roberts I. The healthcare assistant: Professional supported or budget necessity. *Health Manpower Management* 1995; 21(5): 25–37.

Rye D. Nursing auxiliaries: A professional perspective. In: Hardie M, Hockey L. (eds.) *Nursing Auxiliaries in Health Care.* London: Croom Helm; 1978, pp. 65–76.

Saks M, Allsop J. Social policy, professional regulation and health support work in the UK. *Social Policy and Society* 2007; 6(2): 165–77.

Sawada A. The nursing shortage problem in Japan. *Nursing Ethics* 1997; 4(3): 245–52.

Scott C. *Setting safe nurse staffing levels: An exploration of the issues.* London: RCN; 2003.

Selfe J, Roddam H, Cording H, Temple B, Green L, Chambers A. *Assistant Practitioner Evaluation Foundation degree Evaluation Project Final Report.* UK: University of Central Lancashire (UCLAN); 2008.

Simoens S, Villeneuve M, Hurst J. *Tackling nurse shortages in OECD countries.* OECD Working Papers 19. Paris: OECD; 2005.

Skills for Health. *The role of Assistant Practitioners in the NHS: Factors affecting the evolution and development of the role.* Bristol: Skills for Health; 2011.

Skills for Health. *The Thames Gateway Project, Final Report.* Skills for Health [Online] 2009; Available at: http://www.skillsforhealth.org.uk/about-us/resource-library/doc_download/1668-tgp-final-report-160709.html [Accessed 12 December 2011].

Smith P. *The Emotional Labour of Nursing.* Basingstoke: Palgrave Macmillan; 1992.

Snee T. Nursing auxiliaries—training for what? The dilemma of nursing education. In: Hardie M, Hockey L. (eds) *Nursing Auxiliaries in Health Care.* London: Croom Helm; 1978, pp. 77–85.

South African Nursing Council. *Regulations Relating to the Scope of Practice of Persons Who are Registered or Enrolled under the Nursing Act, 1978. Government Notice No. R. 2598.* Pretoria: South African Nursing Council; 1991.

Spilsbury K. 'Who Cares? A case study to explore HCAs' Jurisdiction in a hospital setting.' PhD thesis, City University London; 2004.

Spilsbury K, Meyer J. Defining the nursing contribution to patient outcomes: lessons form a review of the literature examining nursing outcomes, skill mix and changing roles. *Journal of Clinical Nursing* 2001; 10: 3–14.

Spilsbury K, Meyer J. Use, misuse and non use of healthcare assistant: understanding the work of HCAs in a hospital setting. *Journal of Nursing Management* 2004; 12: 411–18.

Spilsbury K, Stuttard L, Adamson J, Atkin K, Borglin G, McCaughan D, McKenna H, Wakefield A, Carr-Hill R. Mapping the introduction of assistant practitioners in acute NHS trusts in England. *Journal of Nursing Management* 2009; 17(5): 615–26.

Statistisches Bundesamt. *Gesundheitspersonal [Health Personnel].* 2010 [Online] Available at: http://www.destatis.de/jetspeed/portal/cms/Sites/destatis/Internet/DE/Content/Statistiken/Gesundheit/Gesundheitspersonal/Tabellen/Content75/Berufe,templateId=renderPrint.psml [Accessed 12 December 2011].

Stokes J, Warden A. The changing role of the healthcare assistant. *Nursing Standard* 2004; 18(51): 33–7.

Sutton J, Valentine J, Rayment K. Staff views on the extended role of health care assistants in the critical care unit. *Intensive and Critical Care Nursing* 2004; 20(5): 249–56.

Temple J. *Time for Training. A Review of the Impact of the European Working Time Directive on the Quality of Training.* London: HMSO; 2010.

The Guardian. Lansley publishes McKinsey report on NHS productivity. *The Guardian* [Online] 2010; 3 June; Available at: http://www.guardian.co.uk/society/interactive/2010/jun/02/mckinsey-report-future-nhs [Accessed 12 December 2011].

The Health and Social Care Information Centre. *NHS Workforce: Summary of Staff in the NHS: Results from September 2010 Census.* Leeds: NHSIHSC; 2011.

The Observer. Paper work mountains keep nurses from care. *The Observer* 2005; 27 November; Available at: http://www.guardian.co.uk/society/2005/nov/27/health.uknews1 [Accessed 12 December 2011].

Theodosius C. *Emotional Labour in Health Care: The Unmanaged Heart of Nursing.* Abingdon: Routledge; 2008.

Thomas L. A comparison of the verbal interaction of qualified nurses and nursing auxiliaries in primary, team and fuctional nursing wards. *International Journal of Nursing Studies* 1994; 31(3): 231–44.

Thornley C. Segmentation and Inequality in the Nursing Workforce. In: Crompton R, Gallie D, Purcell K. (eds.) *Changing Forms of Employment*. London: Routledge; 1996, pp. 160–81.

Thornley C. *The Invisible Workers: Health Care Assistants and Support Workers*. London: UNISON; 1997.

Thornley, C. A question of competence? Re-evaluating the roles of the nursing auxiliary and health care assistant in the NHS. *Journal of Clinical Nursing* 2000; 9: 451–8.

Thornley C. *Double Jeopardy; non-registered nurses in the NHS*. Paper presented to Gender Research Forum, Women's Equality Unit, London, 8 November; 2002.

Tierney MJ, Tierney L. Nursing Japan. *Nursing Outlook* 1994; 42(5): 313–22.

UNISON. *Just a Little Respect*. London: UNISON; 2008.

United Kingdom Central Council for Nursing, Midwifery and Health Visiting. *Project 2000: A New Preparation for Practice*. London: UKCC; 1986.

US Bureau of labor Statistics. *Occupational Outlook Handbook*. US Bureau of Labor Statistics 2011 [Online]; Available at: http://www.bls.gov/oco/ocos327.htm [Accessed 12 December 2011].

Vail L, Bosely S, Petrova M, Dale J. Health care assistants in general practice: a qualitative study of their experience. *Primary Health Care Research and Development* 2010; 12(1): 29–41.

Wainwright T. The perceived function of HCAs in intensive care: nurses views. *Intensive and Critical Care Nursing* 2002; 18(3): 171–80.

Wakefield A, Spilsbury K, Atkin K, McKenna H, Borglin G, Stuttard L. Assistant or substitute: Exploring the fit between national policy vision and local practice realities of assistant practitioner job descriptions, *Health Policy* 2009; 90(2): 286–95.

Wanless D. *Securing Our Future Health Taking a Long Term View*. London: HM Treasury; 2002.

Webb B. Enrolled nurse conversion: A review of the literature. *Journal of Nursing Management* 2000; 8: 115–20.

Workman B. An Investigation into how the health care assistants perceive their role as 'support workers' to qualified staff. *Journal of Advanced Nursing* 1996; 23: 612–19.

Xu Y, Xu Z, Zhang MA. The nursing education system in the People's Republic of China: evolution, structure and reform. *International Nursing Review* 2000; 47(4): 207–17.

Appendix

Table A1 Overview of nurse support role research

	Focus	Country	Method	Findings
Chang (1995)	Professional nurse views on non-nursing duties and possible use of support personnel	Hong Kong	Questionnaire survey, 408 nurse respondents	Three-quarters agree support worker would be useful
Hancock (2006)	Preparedness of HCAs to develop a new role and attend HCA development programme Impact of HCA development programme on role of HCA in one trust on other members of team and patients	UK	Interview study with 12 HCAs	Most HCAs prepared to attend programme. Positive but restricted impact of the development programme on HCA role, other team members and patients
Wainwright (2002)	Nurse views on function of HCAs in ICU	UK	Questionnaire survey in one Trust, 24 out of 25 nurses responded	Strong support for introduction of HCA role, but different views on its use
Meek (1998)	Service user evaluation of the role of HCAs in community mental health intensive care team	UK	Repertory grid/ structured interviews with 14 service users	User satisfaction with HCAs Emphasis on personal qualities of the HCA

(*Continued*)

Table A1 Overview of nurse support role research (Continued)

	Focus	Country	Method	Findings
Ford (2004)	Views of NHS radiology service managers on concept of support workers using ionizing radiations	UK	Group discussion/ questionnaire/ 16 managers in SE England	Widespread agreement on need to train support workers to undertake work using ionizing radiations Differences of view on what cohorts of patient they should be allowed to examine
Jack et al. (2004)	Hospital ward managers' views on current and potential expansion of HCA role	UK	Survey in single trust, 33 respondents	HCAs undertaking wide diversity of procedures. Most managers say role could be expanded, but concern about additional training
McLaughlin et al. (2000)	Comparative study of nurse views on changes in their role when working with assistants Nurse perceptions of assistant to perform delegate duties	UK/USA	Questionnaire survey in three UK trusts. Responses from 171 UK nurses and 216 from the USA	UK nurses have higher satisfaction with assistants than nurses from the USA
Thomas (1994)	Compares differential contribution to patient care of nurses and HCAs in primary, team, and functional nursing wards	UK	12 nurses and 12 HCAs observed and computerized events recorded	Wards practising primary nursing gave patients more choice, general explanations about their care, and spent more time seeking verbal feedback from patients about their care

Table A1 Overview of nurse support role research (Continued)

	Focus	Country	Method	Findings
Furaker (2008)	To describe the work and everyday activities of HCAs and mental attendants in acute hospital care	Sweden	Diary study of 26 HCAs and 10 MAs	Half the time of assistants spent on direct care, but differences between wards
Sutton et al. (2004)	To capture views on HCA role extension in critical care	UK	Audit of 54 staff in a critical care unit in one trust. Changes implemented followed by re-audit	Support for extended HCA role. Consensus on appropriate tasks for HCAs
Perry et al. (2003)	Understanding main differences between roles/functions of nurses and assistants	UK	Interviews with nine nurses and 12 assistants	Nurses report difficulty defining roles. Assistants define roles by what they cannot do. Nurses find delegation difficult. Both staff groups agree assistant role necessary for good quality care
Gould et al. (1996)	Evaluating new systems of nursing care that change nurse and HCA role—working together to care for group of patients	USA	Staff survey three months after change in one hospital	Decrease in overtime and decrease in concerns over care quality
Keeney et al. (2005)	Obtain views of managers of health care agencies to assess whether they would employ trained HCAs	Ireland	Questionnaire survey to health care agencies. 103 managers responded	Suggestions given on more relevant training. Most managers did not feel HCA role encroached on that of the nurse and would employ HCAs trained on the programme

(Continued)

Table A1 Overview of nurse support role research (Continued)

	Focus	Country	Method	Findings
Johnson et al. (2004)	Evaluating the views of a multidisciplinary team on the role of advanced support workers in intensive care settings	UK	Interviews, focus groups, and observation in six intensive care units across Greater Manchester. All 17 senior support workers were interviewed	Senior support workers have a potentially important but as yet insufficiently clear role; concern about accountability; a reluctance to delegate unless personally assessed.
Hogan and Playle (2000)	Identify how HCAs are utilized within general intensive care environment	UK	Questionnaire survey within general intensive care units across the UK; 42 responses (76% response rate)	Wide variation between units in how HCAs used, their training and pay.
Chang and Lam (1998)	Differences in the type and pattern of work performed by student nurses and HCAs	Hong Kong	Non-participant observation in four clinical areas in one hospital	No significant differences found in total amount of all types of activity performed by nurses and HCAs. However, in direct care work HCAs performed more basic care
Grimshaw (1999)	Impact of HCA recruitment on wage inequality amongst nurses. Impact of local HCAs on demarcations between qualified/unqualified staff	UK	Care studies in two Trusts using pay/staffing data and interviews with personnel	Context dependent nature of local pay systems. Evidence of skill mix dilution

Table A1 Overview of nurse support role research (Continued)

	Focus	Country	Method	Findings
Workman (1996)	Method of work allocated to HCAs; main tasks performed by HCAs; how HCAs perceive their role; relationship between nurse and HCA from HCA viewpoint	UK	Eight HCAs from one hospital who had completed at least 15 study days over a one year period were interviewed	Inconclusive results on work allocation. Most common HCA task was tidying up. The HCA–nurse relationship good, but depended on how treated by nurse
Thornley (2000)	The number of HCAs; managerial reasons for introducing HCAs; the HCA role; HCA training; and HCA characteristics	UK	A survey of trust HR managers (n = 80); a national survey of NAs (n = 1031); in-depth interviews with HCAs, managers, and UNISON officers	80% of trusts employing HCAs. Cost effectiveness main reason for introducing the role. Highly blurred nurses/ NA boundaries. NVQs becoming expected. HCAs over 30 years old with considerable caring experience and length of service
Gould et al. (2006)	Role transitions of newly qualified nurses who had been HCAs	UK	Interviews in one Trust with 12 former HCAs plus managers and clinical practice facilitators	HCA secondments may not offer ready solution to increasing qualified nursing workforce. Highlighted HCA difficulties in training

(Continued)

Table A1 Overview of nurse support role research (Continued)

	Focus	Country	Method	Findings
Cox et al. (2008)	How can pay systems improve the prospects for lower skilled workers? How can skills development initiatives facilitate career progression for such workers?	UK	Interviews with HR managers and training staff across 13 Trust cases	One-off improvements in pay following AfC. But uncertainty about sustainability of pay improvements. Career progression opportunities heavily contingent on management strategy in Trust
Spilsbury and Meyer (2004)	Understanding the work of HCAs in a hospital setting	UK	Single hospital case study using mixed methods: interviews (n = 33 HCAs), focus groups and observation (220 hours)	Policy expectations on work of HCA. Practice deviates from these. HCA work shaped by HCA-nurse negotiations. Dynamic pattern of use, non use and misuse of HCAs
Brennan and McSherry (2007)	Determine the transition process associated with moving from HCA to student nurse	UK	Four focus groups covering 14 nurse students with HCA experience	Positive/negative perceptions of process revealed
Knibb et al. (2006)	Exploring the work of nursing assistants in hospital setting	UK	Surveys, interviews, and focus groups with nursing assistants and ward managers in two Trusts	The nursing assistant role varied by clinical area; an urgent need to clarify the role; scope to extend the role
Spilsbury (2009)	The take-up of assistant practitioner roles	UK	Survey of English Trusts	Limited but uneven take-up of assistant practitioner roles

Table A1 Overview of nurse support role research (Continued)

	Focus	**Country**	**Method**	**Findings**
Vail et al. (2010)	Experience of HCAs working in GP practice	UK	Interviews with 14 HCAs from two Primary Care Trusts	HCAs enjoyed role and especially the contact with patients. Views affected by previous work experience and length of service. Some source of frustration around pay

Index